THE CHRONIC FATIGUE HEALING DIET

CHRISTINE CRAGGS-HINTON, mother of three, followed a career in the Civil Service until, in 1991, she developed fibromyalgia. Christine the last few years, produced *Living with Fibromyalgia* and *The Fibromyalgia Healing Diet* (both published by Sheldon Press). She also writes for the Fibromyalgia Association UK and the related *FaMily* magazine. In recent years she has also become interested in fiction writing.

Overcoming Common Problems Series

A full list of titles is available from Sheldon Press,
1 Marylebone Road, London NW1 4DU, and on our website at
www.sheldonpress.co.uk

Overcoming Common Problems Series

Overcoming Common Problems Series

Overcoming Common Problems

The Chronic Fatigue Healing Diet

Christine Craggs-Hinton

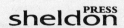

First published in Great Britain in 2003 by
Sheldon Press
1 Marylebone Road
London NW1 4DU

British Library Cataloguing-in-Publication Data

A catalogue record for this book is available from the British Library

ISBN 0–85969–878–5

Typeset by Deltatype Limited, Birkenhead, Merseyside
Printed in Great Britain by Biddles Ltd
www.biddles.co.uk

Contents

This book is dedicated to all the people who live with CFS/ME every day. Many healthy people have little comprehension of this disease – but as the medical profession and the media become slowly enlightened, things are beginning to change. However, until we have that great breakthrough in treatment, improved diet is the best option. Don't curse the darkness – light a candle.

Acknowledgements

I would like to say a special thanks to:

Susan Thorpe, homeopath, holistic adviser, healthfoods expert and my good friend, for her tireless efforts in helping me to produce this book. Susan has been of great assistance at each and every turn, passing on so many articles and information sheets that my office shelves are now bulging under the weight! Without her, this book would not be nearly so thorough.

Steve Taylor, a nutritionist and friend, for carrying out the final and very detailed check on my work and for providing the foreword. His help is much appreciated.

David Craggs-Hinton, my husband, for supporting me in everything I do, for not minding when I sit tapping away at my computer at night and forgetting to talk to him, and for kindly trying out the recipes used in this book. His presence in my life has made anything possible.

Foreword

More and more people are looking towards alternative therapies after receiving little help from orthodox medicine. This has launched a myriad of therapies, supplements, superfoods, miracle cures, etc. As with the orthodox, some people benefit, but there are many who end up clutching at straws and trying anything going. I am not advising people not to go to their doctor or their alternative therapist, but instead, to be aware that one person's miracle cure is not necessarily right for another.

However, nutrition is fundamental to optimum health. By this I really do mean fundamental. If you don't take a prescribed drug you probably will not die. If you don't have acupuncture you probably will not die. If you don't take the latest 'snake oil' you will probably not die. However, if you don't take nutrition, i.e. water, carbohydrates, proteins, fats, minerals and vitamins, you will die. Therefore nutrition, quite literally, is fundamental to survival.

In my work as a nutrition consultant I have many stories of amazing improvements in client symptoms just by correcting fundamental areas of their nutrition. ME is a multi-faceted complaint and there have been times when a nutritional approach has not been the total answer. Homeopathy, Reiki and meditation, acupuncture have all worked for different individuals. However, I have not come across anyone who has tried a nutritional approach and said that it has had no benefit at all. The essence of Christine Craggs-Hinton's book has come from her own experiences with ME/fibromyalgia and revolves around foods that are unadulterated, organic and wholesome. Fundamental. I think you will benefit from reading this book.

Steve Taylor
BANT (British Association of Nutritional Therapists)

Introduction

It's a sad fact that conventional medications merely treat the symptoms of CFS/ME (chronic fatigue syndrome/myalgic encephalomyelitis) rather than addressing the underlying problems. Maybe one day scientists will find a cure – a pill or a potion that will miraculously energize sufferers, end the aching, poor sleep, memory and concentration problems, food and chemical intolerances and everything else. However, until that day arrives, the best option is a little less straightforward and demands a lot more effort. It is the best option, though. What is it? A tailor-made diet.

Food is actually the finest medicine we can put into our bodies and is the best means of influencing health. Not only does food keep us alive, it also works to repair and regenerate the tissues, warding off further disease and allowing a longer, more fruitful life. There is no doubt that powerful medicines and treatments are invaluable in a life-threatening situation, for correcting congenital abnormality and so on, but, unfortunately, using drugs to suppress long-standing symptoms is merely a temporary solution.

Because certain foods act on certain parts of the body, it has been possible to devise a diet that targets the problem areas in CFS/ME. Consequently, this book describes the foods that help to strengthen the immune, endocrine and central nervous systems. It also explains how to overcome the food intolerances and toxic build-up that are perhaps universal in CFS/ME. The nutritional supplements known to be beneficial in treating the condition are also outlined, as is the important 21-day detoxification programme.

Now read on, go shopping – or ask someone to do it for you – then get on with helping your body to begin healing itself! If making more than modest dietary changes is difficult at this early stage, remember that every little thing you do helps and, as you improve, you should be able to invest more and more energy into planning and cooking your meals.

Stay close to nature, and its eternal laws will protect you
Dr Max Gerson

Note The diet described in this book should only be followed with your doctor's approval. The author is not able to independently dispense medical advice, nor can she prescribe remedies or assume any responsibility for those who treat themselves without the consent of their doctor. As some nutritional supplements may interact with certain medicines, and as they may adversely affect particular medical conditions, please consult your doctor before embarking on a course.

PART ONE

1

What it Means to Suffer from CFS/ME

No one really knows how long CFS/ME has been around. Some believe it was described in the Bible as the 'afflictions of Job', others that it was actually the 'muscular rheumatism' reported in the 1680s. It even seems that Florence Nightingale and Charles Darwin may have been nineteenth-century victims. However, it was not until the 1930s that epidemics began to occur, and with increasing regularity. Nowadays, we know that large numbers of people – an estimated 2–3 per cent of the population – are affected by this mysterious malaise. So what exactly is it?

Symptoms

People with CFS/ME live every day with symptoms that mimic a bad dose of the flu. These symptoms may include fatigue to the point of extreme exhaustion, aching muscles and joints, sweating and shivering, a poor sleep pattern, headaches, tender lymph nodes in the neck, problems with memory and concentration, loss of balance, tinnitus and sensitivity to light. Victims are also likely to suffer from food and chemical sensitivities, poor thyroid and adrenal function, poor blood sugar control and chronic yeast infections (all of these are described in Chapter 7).

To complicate matters further, CFS/ME is a disease that affects people differently. Some will experience symptoms so severe that they are confined to bed, while others may encounter symptoms only when faced with stressful situations. The course of the disease will often wax and wane, too – worsening when provoked by overactivity, anxiety or for no apparent reason. In some cases, symptoms may even disappear altogether, although this occurs all too rarely.

Possible causes

The causes of CFS/ME are not clear, but scientists have found evidence that the disease is related to a virus, which is supported by the fact that flu-like symptoms are experienced. Interestingly, signs of persistent enterovirus infections have been found by researchers in about 60 per cent of sufferers. These infections are believed to be mutated forms of a poliovirus that attack the brain, causing a 'cascade effect' of symptoms. Many more viruses are under investigation.

Researchers have also discovered signs of abnormality in the central nervous system (located in the brain and spinal cord) of people with CFS/ME. They have found evidence of deregulated hormone activity, too. There are also ample indications of immune system disturbance. Parts of the immune system are known to be overactive, giving rise to autoimmune problems (when the immune system begins to attack the body's own tissues) and other parts have been found to be underactive, leaving the body vulnerable to attack.

Furthermore, an abnormal protein has been detected in the natural antiviral defence mechanisms of sufferers. It is estimated that a third of patients diagnosed with CFS/ME have too much of this protein – called 37 kDa RnaseL – yet what they do have is underdeveloped and less able to protect them against viruses. As a result, viruses are weakened but not killed, resulting in ongoing problems.

Experts now commonly acknowledge that people with CFS/ME are affected adversely by environmental factors, too. Sufferers are believed to poorly tolerate biological stressors and, as a result, have difficulty eliminating toxins from their bodies. This results in toxic overload. In fact, people with CFS/ME have been likened to human canaries, for most are sensitive to all manner of environmental pollutants, much as canaries are to gases. It could be said, then, that, as canaries were to mineworkers, CFS/ME sufferers are the signal to the rest of the population that our world is becoming hazardous.

Because the condition is lacking in defining structural defects, diagnosis is notoriously difficult. As a consequence, routine laboratory tests often come back 'normal', which is not the relief you might assume it to be. Unfortunately, until researchers find definitive evidence of the presence of disease, the medical profession and media may continue to view CFS/ME with scepticism – a situation that causes sufferers a great deal of upset.

It may interest you to know that the cause of chronic illness is now starting to be viewed in a different light. Scientists have been accustomed to looking at all the individual parts of complex bodily systems in an effort to learn how it all works. They had hoped that, in this way, they would learn how systems malfunction in those with disease. However, they are now realizing that understanding the individual parts will not necessarily reveal what they wish to know. Complex systems require an additional 'emergent property' that can only be seen when all the parts are working together (networking). Think of a flock of birds in flight and you will have a good idea of what this means. The way the flock acts as one is an emergent property that cannot be known by looking at individual birds alone. This explains why the exact cause of CFS/ME is so difficult to pinpoint.

It does appear, however, that the disease may arise because some of the body's control systems set themselves wrongly, giving rise to network errors – that is, the way the body's systems communicate with each other is malfunctioning. It seems that the errors occur in the first place because of a lifestyle problem, such as an infection, too much stress, toxic overload and/or overactivity.

The benefits of an improved diet

As CFS/ME is a disease in which the balance of the body is clearly affected, the immune system should be supported by working from every angle possible to help the body back into balance. When, as a result, the bodily systems are once again networking properly, the errors will begin to correct themselves. The most vital area of support is improved nutrition for, among its many benefits, it is of enormous help to the body at the important cellular level.

Cell health

The human body is capable of complete rejuvenation, regeneration and repair. In other words, it can heal itself, given the right conditions, mentally and physically. Good nutrition is the most vital factor in establishing good physical health. This is because it allows our cells – the smallest but most important components in our bodies – to be nourished continuously and washed clean of waste. Our cells do not function at their optimum levels if they are seldom fed and cleansed. In fact, poor nutrition diminishes cell function, causes gradual toxic build-up within the cells, triggers disease and exacerbates the ageing process.

Although we have much to eat in the West, quite a lot of food has frighteningly little nutritional value. This happens because it is grown in overused soils that are loaded with harmful chemicals and lack essential minerals. Needing a boost of energy, we turn to stimulants such as coffee, sugar, junk food and alcohol. However, these are actually toxic substances that make the liver hyperactive in its attempt to filter out the toxins. This, in turn, speeds up the metabolism, demanding a short, yet intense energy capacity that is stolen from the cells and the immune system. As a result, the body feels fatigued. The longer this cycle continues as a result of a harmful diet, the more fatigued the body becomes, at the cellular level.

This situation – called 'acidosis' – is reflected in the individual's mental, physical and emotional makeup. It creates a seriously ineffective immune system and a body that is struggling to run on empty. The acidosis causes imbalances within the organs, the digestive tract and the cells, allowing parasites, unfriendly bacteria, fungi and viruses to take over. Improved nutrition is the only answer.

Our cells are being replaced constantly on a rotational basis. With the correct help (see below) each unhealthy old cell can be replaced by a healthy new one, leading to better, total health. However, this does take time. Think of a neglected houseplant which you start feeding and watering appropriately. The leaves perk up a bit from the improved nutrition, but you have to wait for the old leaves to die off and the new ones to grow before you have a truly healthy plant. It is the same with the human body. When you start feeding and treating it better, you have to wait for the physiological dynamics of the body to grow new improved cells in every area.

I must add that when good nutrition – together with exercise, fresh air and a reduction in stress – fails to bring about positive changes in health, it may be useful to see a registered homeopath. Homeopathy is entirely natural and aims to stimulate the body's own healing forces. This therapy can be used to complement your doctor's treatment and advice without causing an adverse reaction, but if you do decide to see a homeopath, make sure that your doctor is aware of this.

How it used to be

There have been few changes to our bodies – in a genetic or physiological sense – since the days of the ancient hunter–gatherer. Our basic foodstuffs are very similar, too. What have changed, dramatically, are our lifestyle, behaviour and diet – the latter having altered a great deal since World War II. Nature takes a long time to make changes, whereas humans can make radical shifts within a generation or two. This is much too fast for our bodies to adjust to.

Our diet today consists largely of processed foods – that is, foods grown on land laden with chemicals and containing chemical preservatives, flavourings and colourings. We generally consume our foods in a stressful environment, too, whereas cave-dwellers undoubtedly had lots of time to relax. Their foods were not sprayed with chemicals, they did not contain preservatives. Instead, they were eaten fresh and in season – and fresh, uncontaminated fruit and vegetables are highly nutritious. They are also rich in enzymes – the substances that aid digestion. For the most part, their food was uncooked, too. Unfortunately, cooking above 41°C (107°F) and refrigeration destroy live digestive enzymes that help to break down food.

Cave-dwellers would no doubt have enjoyed variety, but they would certainly not have had the opportunity to combine as many foods in one sitting as we do today. When they came to an apple tree, they probably sat down and ate only apples. They also ate their food whole – not just the tasty parts, as is the present custom. As a result, they consumed a great deal of fibre – the roughage that ensures regular and efficient bowel function. In contrast, modern man's elimination of waste product from the body is dreadful. The passage of chyme (partially digested food) through the bowel is very slow and so the body is susceptible to debris and waste accumulation. This causes the reabsorption of toxins and waste matter into the body.

Because cave-dwellers consumed freshly gathered, uncontaminated 'whole' foods, however, their digestive systems would have functioned superbly. They also had the benefit of fresh air and exercise contributing to their good health. It is doubtful that our ancient ancestors developed CFS/ME.

Foodstuffs today

Nowadays, the average Western diet is very poor. It is estimated that we eat approximately 17 per cent of our daily calories as processed foods, 18 per cent as saturated fats, 18 per cent as sugar and 3–10 per cent as alcoholic beverages. When you add this up, more than half of our foods are high in calories and low in nutrients. It is little wonder, then, that, over time, many of us develop chronic disease.

Here is an outline of current food habits.

• We eat food grown on artificially fertilized land and sprayed many times with chemical pesticides, herbicides and fungicides. These poisons kill essential soil microbes that would otherwise help plants to absorb nutrient-rich minerals that are essential to good health.

- Plant foods are then artificially ripened, stored and processed. Unfortunately, the refining and storage process robs food of the majority of its fibre and nutrients. Most of the precious B vitamins and vitamin E are lost in the processing of wheat and flour, leaving it valueless and literally poisonous to the body. Similarly, all other cereals, fruits and vegetables lose their nutrients and vitamin C during processing.
- We eat the tasty parts of the food only, disposing of the rest. For example, wheat husks and wheatgerm – the most nutritious parts of the plant – are removed before the remaining cereal is processed into white flour. 'Whole' foods contain fibre and so aid the removal of waste materials from the bowel. They are vital to good bowel health.
- We prefer taste to quality.
- We grow foods from hybrid seeds.
- We eat hurriedly, often while working or thinking about problems.
- We dilute the nutrients in our food by drinking at the same time.

The symptoms of CFS/ME can be improved considerably if we get back to basics in terms of our diet. The highly processed, flavoured, coloured foods we can consume without thinking may seem fine but are not helping us to get well at all. In the next chapter we will see what kinds of changes we can make to help ourselves – changes for the better in all senses.

2

Beginning to Make Changes for the Better

Changing the habits of a lifetime takes a lot of effort and determination. Eating is a pleasurable activity and we are used to choosing the foods that satisfy our taste buds – often made more tasty by the addition of chemical flavourings, fat, sugar, salt and so on – and may be loath to make drastic changes. For these reasons, I recommend that you alter your eating habits gradually, allowing yourself time to adjust to the new textures, appearance and flavours of different foods. With perseverance, your tastes will change and, as your CFS/ME symptoms gradually decline, your interest in the new diet will likely increase.

If you wish to start eating the new foods straightaway, I must add a word of warning, however. Nutritious, cleanly grown foods may trigger the body into instant detoxification, causing headaches, lethargy and even diarrhoea, lasting between one day and two weeks. You can avoid this shock to your body by changing over to better foods very gradually.

When starting to introduce the new diet, remember that it is important to eat a wide variety of foods. To eat the same things repeatedly means missing out on many vital building blocks of life, for certain foods build and regenerate only certain parts of the body. Eating the same foods can also lead to food sensitivities and allergies. Because people with CFS/ME don't tolerate toxins and pollutants well, it is necessary to eat an organic diet with plenty of fresh fruit and vegetables and look for foods without added chemicals (colourings, flavourings, preservatives and so on). A diet that is free of immunosuppressants (substances that suppress the immune system), such as coffee and alcohol, is also recommended. I reiterate that it is important to eat whole foods, too.

A whole food diet

Whole foods are simply those that have had nothing taken away – that is, nutrients and fibre – and have had nothing added – colourings, flavourings, preservatives. In short, they are foods in their most natural form. Whole foods that are organically produced – without the use of potentially dangerous chemical fertilizers, pesticides and herbicides – are even better for us than other whole foods.

If your symptoms make it difficult for you to cook in the conventional way, an exciting array of organic convenience foods using whole food ingredients is now available in some supermarkets and healthfood shops.

Let us take a brief look at the main building blocks of the diet that will help your body.

Fresh fruit and vegetables

Because there is likely to be acid buildup in the tissues of CFS/ME sufferers, much of the diet recommended consists of alkalizing foods, which help to reduce acid in the body. Fruit and vegetables are alkaline. Try to eat locally grown, organic foods that are in season. They have the highest levels of nutrients and the greatest enzyme activity. Enzymes are to our body what spark plugs are to the car engine. Without its 'sparks', the body doesn't work properly. Organically grown fruit and vegetables may not look as perfect as those that are processed, but they are superior as processed foods have been devitalized of their 'sparks'.

Try to eat fruit and vegetables as fresh and as raw as possible. Make a variety of salads during the course of a week and try to eat one every day. When you do cook vegetables, cook them in the minimum of unsalted (or lightly salted) water for the minimum of time. Lightly steaming or stir-frying are healthy alternatives. Scrub rather than peel.

Pulses

Although they contain high levels of protein, pulses cost very little. The soya bean is a complete protein and there are many soya bean products, including soya milk, tofu, tempeh and miso. Tofu, for example, is very versatile and can be used in both savoury and sweet dishes.

Seeds

They are not only for the birds. Sunflower, sesame, hemp and pumpkin seeds contain a wonderful combination of nutrients – all necessary to start a new plant – and so are very important to the healing process. They can be eaten as they are as a snack, sprinkled on to salads and cereals or used in baking. For more flavour, they can be lightly roasted and coated with organic soy sauce or Herbamare seasoning (see the Useful Addresses section at the back of this book for details of a supplier of the latter). Cracked linseeds are also highly nutritious and useful for treating constipation. Linseed can be used in baking and sprinkled on to breakfast cereals and porridge oats.

Nuts

Nuts, too, are an intrinsic part of this diet. All nuts contain vital nutrients, but almonds, cashews, walnuts, Brazils and pecans perhaps offer the greatest array. Eat a wide assortment of unsalted, uncoated nuts as snacks, with cereal and in baking.

Grains

Whole grains and wholemeal flours provide us with the complex unrefined carbohydrates our bodies require – again, organic is best. There are many types of grains, but wheat is our staple in the West. It is found in most breads, cakes, pastries, biscuits and so on. Although nutritious, wheat is an acid food that is not recommended for people with CFS/ME as the body may be overly acidic already – due to the condition acidosis, mentioned earlier. Containing gluten, it is also the number two food allergen (after dairy products), causing some sufferers to have adverse reactions to it.

Aim to consume a variety of grains, including oats, rye, barley (generally available as pearl barley), corn, buckwheat, brown rice and mixed grains. Millet is highly recommended for people with CFS/ME as it is an alkaline food that helps to reduce acidosis. Oats are important, too, as they help to stabilize blood sugar levels. Brown rice, millet, buckwheat and maize/corn are all gluten-free and invaluable to people with a gluten allergy or sensitivity.

Reducing sugar

An important aspect of the chronic fatigue healing diet is limited consumption of sugar and salt. Sugar – which has been dubbed 'the scourge of the age' – has no nutritional value at all. In fact, sugar consumption has been linked with many disorders, from diabetes to heart disease and cancer. It also exacerbates the chronic candida (yeast) problem so common in people with CFS/ME (more information about candida in Chapter 7).

You probably know that sugar is converted by the body into energy. What you may not know is that we can actually obtain all the sugars and energy we need from fruit and complex (unrefined) carbohydrates (grains, lentils and so on), which are converted into sugar in the body in the way nature intended.

Reducing salt

Salt is commonly used as a preservative and added to most processed, prepackaged foods – cornflakes, for example, are high in salt. As a result, people who eat a lot of these types of foods may be consuming more salt than they realize, especially when that used in cooking and at the table is taken into account. However, whole foods actually contain salt (sodium) and potassium in just the right amounts for our bodies. Extra salt upsets this happy balance and can lead to a variety of problems. Try using herbs and spices for flavouring (in moderation) or Bioforce seasonings (see the Useful Addresses section at the back of this book for Bioforce's contact details). Sea salt contains more minerals than ordinary salt, but is still salt, so use it sparingly.

Retraining your palate

In comparison with the average Western diet, which has, by the addition of chemical flavourings, saturated fat, sugar, salt and so on, evolved largely to please the taste buds, the chronic fatigue healing diet is based on foods in their more natural form. It is essential, therefore, that you slowly retrain your palate to accept different tastes. For this reason, it is advisable to cut back gradually on the amounts of sugar, salt and saturated fat you consume. It takes only 28 days of eating a food regularly for it to become a habit.

Keeping a diary

Keeping a food intake diary is an excellent way to monitor your progress. I suggest that you buy a notebook and devote a page to each day, listing all the foods you eat – including snacks and drinks.

Goals

It's a good idea to set goals on the very first page. For example, you may wish to make a goal of eating two types of vegetables each day. Without the diary, you may assume you've done badly, but, on reading your entries, you may see that you've actually eaten two types of vegetables three or four times a week. That's a good starting point. Now you can focus on slowly increasing that amount.

As time goes by and you begin to achieve your goals as a matter of habit, list a new set of slightly more difficult ones. Here are some examples of long-term goals.

- To eat two to three types of vegetables every day – some of them raw.

- To eat two to three portions of fruit every day.
- To eat only whole foods – whole wheat, corn, barley, brown rice and so on.
- To eat nuts, seeds and/or dried fruit as snacks once or twice a day.
- To drink eight to ten glasses of clean water daily, including that in fruit/vegetable juices and herbal teas (see Chapter 8 for further information on drinking water).
- To buy only organically grown produce.
- To use vegetable, corn or olive oils in cooking and dressings. Extra virgin olive oil is best. Hemp oil, which is very nutritious, is great, too, for dressings.
- To minimize the amount of salt added to cooking and baking.
- To reduce intakes of meat and dairy products, making sure to spread butter thinly.
- To avoid heating foods in a microwave oven.
- To avoid sprinkling table salt on food. (If you can't bear to go without salt, use small amounts of sea or rock salt instead.)
- To cut out caffeine – coffee, chocolate, cola drinks, tea and cocoa.
- To cut out junk food.
- To cut out alcohol.
- To cut out table sugar and other products containing sugar, such as cakes, sweets, biscuits, sugar-coated cereals and so on.
- To cut out saturated fats.
- To cut out refined white flour.
- To cut out artificial sweeteners.
- To avoid foods containing additives, preservatives, colourings and so on.
- To cut out fried foods. (Stir-fried food is acceptable, however. Cook in a little water and drizzle on a little olive oil before serving.)

The reasons for minimizing intakes of many of the above foods or cutting them out altogether are explained in later chapters. I will just add that if you are ultimately unable to entirely eliminate certain foods, don't be discouraged. Reducing your intake will decrease the strain on your digestive system and detoxification organs (the liver and kidneys), making a difference to your health.

A symptom column

When marking up your diary pages, it is important to include a symptom column at the end of each week. Although this depends on your own particular symptoms, it could include average energy levels, pain levels, sore lymph nodes, headaches or migraines, stiffness, aching joints, mood, sleep quality, stomach problems, cold hands and feet, general tiredness, concentration, short-term memory and stress levels. Each entry should be marked on a scale of one to ten, with the lower numbers being the least intensity and the higher numbers being greater intensity. This should show improvements that may otherwise be overlooked.

Making essential dietary changes

Although many of the dietary changes necessary are mentioned above, I would like to end this chapter with guidelines that are the foundation of the chronic fatigue healing diet. Remember to make changes gradually.

- Eat one biscuit instead of two and cut yourself a smaller slice of cake prior to eliminating or minimizing foods containing sugar. If you find you are craving sugar, remember that the lift it offers will be brief – the next effect being a plummet into a low mood. Staving off hunger with fruit (fresh and dried), nuts and seeds is not only a far healthier choice, it also stabilizes blood sugar levels, helping to ward off the low mood. (See Chapter 5 for more information on sugar and artificial sweeteners, and the Useful Addresses section at the back of this book for details of a product that helps to diminish cravings for sweet foods.)
- Try to slowly replace products made from white, refined flour with those made from whole grain flours, using only whole grain flours in cooking and baking.
- Reduce your intake of caffeine products very gradually. Withdrawing too fast may cause fatigue and headaches (see Chapter 5 for more information).
- Minimize alcohol consumption prior to complete elimination, particularly if you have symptoms of alcohol intolerance (see Chapter 5 for more information). Please seek your doctor's advice if this is a problem.
- If you smoke, try to stop. It is harmful for many reasons, particularly in CFS/ME (again, see Chapter 5 for information, and the Useful Addresses section for a product that helps to reduce the craving for cigarettes).
- Make shopping lists and buy only what is on them. This will help to reduce any impulse to buy processed foods.

- Stock fresh foods.
- Get into the habit of snacking on a variety of unsalted, uncoated nuts, such as almonds, cashews, walnuts, Brazils and pecans, dried fruit, such as raisins, dates and apricots, and seeds, such as pumpkin, hemp, sesame and sunflower. These should not spoil your appetite for your meal. Obviously, if you suffer from a nut allergy, leave nuts alone.
- Select a salad instead of chips when eating out.
- Get into the habit of drinking fruit juice instead of carbonated drinks. Fruit juices generally satisfy a sweet tooth and can be diluted with water to go further. People with chronic yeast infections (candida), however, should not drink too much fruit juice (see Chapter 7 for more information on candida).
- Slowly increase the number and variety of fruits and vegetables you use.
- Gradually reduce the amount of salt you add to your food and in cooking. Remember that salt is commonly used as a preservative and added to most processed, prepackaged foods. Rock salt, sea salt and Bioforce seasonings are healthier alternatives, but should still be used sparingly. (Bioforce seasonings are available from healthfood shops or from the address in the Useful Addresses section at the back of this book.)
- Wash fruit and vegetables thoroughly before use. If you do buy produce that is not organically grown, remember that it will have been sprayed liberally with pesticides.
- Eat three or four small meals a day, with snacks in between.
- Never go more than two to three hours without eating, which means you should never go hungry. This will help to control your blood sugar levels.
- Don't skip breakfast. After fasting during the night, the body requires the glucose obtained from foods. Studies have shown that when nourishment is withheld, brain function can be compromised.
- Avoid missing a meal. When we allow ourselves to become very hungry, the sugary, high-fat foods that are bad for us become more tempting.
- Listen to your body. Stop eating when you feel satiated. Overeating creates a large mass of food to be digested, overloading the system, causing many associated problems.
- Don't mistake thirst for hunger. As the body's thirst mechanism is poorly developed, determine if you really are hungry – you might simply need a drink instead.

- Don't use your stomach as an emotional rubbish bin. Try to find other outlets for your feelings, such as yoga, Pilates and tai chi, or try seeing a counsellor.
- Relax for at least ten minutes before starting each meal. Also, linger a while afterwards – don't rush off straight after eating.
- Eat unhurriedly and chew thoroughly. Enjoy your food.
- At least half your calorie intake should consist of 'complex' carbohydrates. These include fruit, vegetables and whole grains, such as bulgar wheat, couscous, millet, barley, brown rice and whole wheat (see Chapter 3 for more information).
- Fats (oils) should comprise approximately 25 per cent of your calorie intake. Unsaturated fats (also known as polyunsaturated fats) are greatly beneficial to health. These include olive, safflower, sunflower and corn oils. Saturated fats, however, are largely derived from animals and should be consumed in moderation, if at all. Examples are lard, suet, butter and dripping (see Chapter 3 for more information).
- Protein should make up approximately 25 per cent of your total calorie intake. Sources include organic, free-range chicken, turkey, fish, beans, nuts, seeds and pulses.
- Eat plenty of fibre in the form of fruits, vegetables, whole grain breads, cereals and pulses (see Chapter 3 for more information).
- Junk and fast foods are loaded with harmful additives. Avoid them if at all possible.
- Look out for additives on food labels. Flavourings, colourings and preservatives are often given as E numbers in the ingredients listing. Try to keep your intake of these as low as possible.
- Try not to shop when you feel hungry – you will be less tempted to buy the wrong foods.
- Read labels to ensure that tins, bottles and packets contain only whole food ingredients – nothing added and nothing taken away.
- Avoid refined and processed foods. Those that come in tins, jars and packets almost certainly contain additives (except for most foods purchased in healthfood shops). Fresh foods, on the other hand, are usually additive-free.
- Avoid drinking for at least half an hour before and half an hour after eating. Liquid dilutes the nutritional value of our food.
- Due to the high fibre content of the chronic fatigue healing diet, try to drink eight to ten glasses of water a day, inclusive of fruit and vegetable juices and herbal teas. Distilled or filtered water is highly recommended (see Chapter 6 for more information).
- Take digestive enzymes – in supplement form – if you wish.

Because they aid the production of natural digestive enzymes, they are useful when introducing a high-fibre diet to a stomach fed on junk food for years. Digestive enzymes not only help to reduce flatulence and bloating, they also aid the absorption of nutrients from the foods you eat.

- Take the recommended vitamin and mineral supplements. Because people with CFS/ME suffer many nutritional deficiencies, supplements – tablet-form concentrates of a particular vitamin, mineral and so on – are essential (see Chapter 4 for more information).
- Try to find your therapeutic window of exercise – too little is damaging, as is too much – then follow a regular routine. I know it is incredibly difficult to find the right level of exercise, but once you have done so, the benefits can be great.
- As stress causes damage to the immune system, try your best to avoid it. Speak to the people around you and let them know how stress worsens your condition. Get together with others to solve problems. Do whatever you can to reduce the stress in your life.
- Pace yourself carefully throughout the day. Avoid pushing yourself too hard.
- Look closely at your environment. The way you were living before you developed CFS/ME clearly wasn't good for you, so you may need to change one or two things. Investigate sources of indoor air pollution, including scented products, household cleaners, tobacco smoke, gas appliances, ventilation systems, office machines, construction materials (varnish, paint and so on). Remove suspected triggering agents one at a time and observe the results (see Chapter 8 for more information).

This book describes the recommended diet for people with CFS/ME, including the supplements known to be useful in treating the condition. It also outlines, in Chapter 6, the 21-day detoxification programme that will help your body to eliminate stored toxins and debris. However, I reiterate that it is best to become accustomed to the new foods before embarking on the detoxification programme. Also, let your doctor know that you are going to do this.

3

Healing Foods

Protein, carbohydrates, fat and fibre are essential nutrients that provide our bodies with vital energy. As our bodies are in a constant state of regeneration, they also serve as fundamental building materials. Vitamins and minerals are of almost equal importance and will be discussed in Chapter 5.

As mentioned earlier, junk food, or fast food as it is also called, is not recommended for people with CFS/ME – nor for healthy people for that matter. People can survive on junk food for a while because it is mainly comprised of carbohydrates and fat, which means it has a high energy value. However, because junk food is short of sustaining nutrients, the body will not be able to continue to repair and regenerate indefinitely. It slowly becomes clogged up, like a cog wheel fed treacle instead of oil.

The World Health Organization recommends that we consume five portions of fruit and five portions of vegetables a day. As this is a lot to most people, I suggest trying to eat at least five helpings altogether a day. Each of the following is equivalent to one portion:

- 100 g (4 oz) of a very large fruit, such as watermelon, other varieties of melon or pineapple;
- one large fruit, such as an orange, banana or apple;
- two medium-sized fruits, such as kiwi fruit, plums or satsumas;
- 100 ml ($3\frac{1}{2}$ fl oz) freshly squeezed fruit or vegetable juice;
- 100 g (4 oz) berries or cherries;
- a large bowl of salad;
- 90 g ($3\frac{1}{2}$ oz), cooked weight, green vegetables;
- 80 g ($3\frac{1}{4}$ oz), cooked weight, root vegetables such as carrot, swede (don't include potatoes, sweet potatoes and yams);
- 70 g (3 oz), cooked weight, small vegetables, such as peas and sweetcorn;
- 80 g ($3\frac{1}{4}$ oz) pulses, such as lentils.

Protein

Our bodies are largely constructed of protein and, because the cells, enzymes, immune system and connective tissues are all protein-based, a good, steady supply of this food substance is vital. People

18

with poor muscle strength, food intolerances and abnormal immune systems are likely to be consuming a diet low in protein. In fact, many experts are now linking CFS/ME with inadequate protein intake.

Animal protein – meat, chicken, fish, dairy produce and eggs – contains all the essential amino acids and is one of the few sources of vitamin B12. Unfortunately, animal protein contains no fibre, which is an essential ingredient in the chronic fatigue healing diet. Instead, it can be loaded with saturated fat and cholesterol, which can promote cholesterol-related disease. Consequently, only a small amount of animal protein – excluding oily fish – should be consumed. But for a couple of exceptions (see below), the same applies to dairy products, too.

CFS/ME-friendly sources of protein are lean red meat, poultry, fish, soya products, cottage cheese, organic live yogurt, seeds, nuts and pulses. Look for organic, free-range meat as the pesticides, antibiotics and hormones otherwise used in animal husbandry will have an adverse effect on your health. In a week, a serving of meat or fish no larger than the palm of your hand should be eaten on two or three occasions; two to three organic, free-range eggs should be consumed and butter should be spread very thinly on your wholemeal bread and rye crispbreads. In place of cows' milk, use soya milk (calcium-enriched, if possible), which is rich in protein, or rice milk, which has a high carbohydrate content. Goat's milk is an acceptable alternative, too, and is less likely to cause allergy problems than cows' milk.

Although fruit and vegetables are rich in fibre, carbohydrates and certain vitamins and minerals, they are low in protein. Nuts, seeds and pulses are excellent sources of protein, but must be eaten daily to ensure that you get a full range of amino acids. We need 22 amino acids at the same time and in the right quantity for protein synthesis. If just one is regularly omitted, the synthesis of protein will be greatly limited. It may even cease altogether. We have, therefore, an important reason for consuming sufficient protein-containing foods.

People who eat a lot of grain products (bread, pasta, rice, cereals and so on) are likely to be consuming insufficient protein. This can lead to further weakening of the immune system, which is the last thing you want. When protein intake is low, the body may pull protein from the muscles, which causes further weakness, low energy, low stamina, poor resistance to infection, depression and slow healing of wounds. Protein deficiency symptoms are now being linked with CFS/ME.

Recommended protein consumption

An interesting study into the effects of different quantities of protein intake was conducted in 2000.[1] It showed, surprisingly, that a high-protein diet can improve antioxidant status (read how important antioxidants are in Chapter 4). However, we now know that a very high intake of protein may cause the tissues to be overly acidic, which can promote degenerative disease. Acidosis (too much acid in the body) is virtually universal in CFS/ME. I would advise, therefore, that approximately 25 per cent of your total daily calories consist of protein.

I know it is difficult to judge the exact percentage of a particular food in your diet. However, if you make an effort to consume the recommended amounts of meat, as well as fruit, vegetables, nuts, seeds, pulses, soft-boiled egg yolks, soya products and so on, you will be in the right region. Remember, too, that healing changes should come about even if you are not able to follow this diet to the letter. Try to do the best you can and appreciate the fact that you are helping your body to fight this disease. If you are unable to eat the recommended amounts of protein, I strongly recommend that you take free-form amino acids, which are available from healthfood shops. The 'healthy bacteria' acidophilus is also useful, taken twice a day.

Although I do not advocate counting calories in the chronic fatigue healing diet, the following calorific values should give you a rough idea of not only your protein intake, but also of your total consumption (examples of calories of carbohydrates and fat are given later in this chapter). Depending on your levels of activity, you should be eating between 1800 and 3000 calories a day.

Here are the calorific contents of some common protein foods:

- 28 g (1 oz) of grilled haddock – a very small piece – gives you 40 calories;
- 28 g (1 oz) of roast chicken – also a very small piece – gives you 40 calories;
- 28 g (1 oz) of cottage cheese gives you 15 calories;
- 28 g (1 oz) of Parmesan cheese, 120 calories;
- 28 g (1 oz) of soya beans, 50 calories.
- 28 g (1 oz) of butter, 226 calories (to reiterate, butter should be used very sparingly).

Soya foods

The early onset of osteoporosis – particularly among post-menopausal women – is common in people who, for whatever reason, take little exercise. However, because soya foods are believed to contain plant oestrogens – oestrogen being one of the hormones that are in short supply during and after the menopause – they are a useful addition to the diet. Not only do soya foods help to limit bone density loss, they also assist in reducing hot flushes, irritability, aching joints and depression, all of which are menopausal symptoms. One study[2] showed that a group of post-menopausal women who consumed more foods containing soya than another group had increased bone mass, fewer backaches and aching joints.

There is a drawback, however. Although rich in protein and very nutritious, soya acts as a hormone in the body and can interact with the delicate balance of thyroxine – the hormone produced by the thyroid gland. High levels of consumption of soya products can suppress thyroid function, causing hypothyroidism (the state where thyroid levels are consistently too low). Pre-existing hypothyroidism may also be worsened.

I would advise, then, that you drink no more than one glass of soya milk a day, maybe having a glass of rice milk later on if you feel like having more milk. Other soya products, such as tofu, tempeh, miso and boiled soya beans, should be eaten once every other day.

For women, wild yam helps to prevent osteoporosis and menopausal symptoms, as do natural progesterone creams that are rubbed into the skin (see the Further Reading section for details of a book that deals with the prevention of menopausal symptoms and osteoporosis).

Carbohydrates

Our digestive systems break down carbohydrates into simple sugars that are used to fuel essential bodily processes, such as the functioning of the brain, nervous system and muscles. In short, we obtain vital energy from foods that contain carbohydrates. A word of warning, however – any excess carbohydrate is converted into fat by insulin, the 'fat-storage' hormone.

To ensure that fats and proteins are broken down effectively and guarantee the production of sufficient energy, we need to eat plenty of complex carbohydrates. These include fruit, vegetables and grains (wholemeal bread, pasta, brown rice, cereals, couscous, millet, barley, bulgar wheat and other cereals). Simple carbohydrates can be detrimental to health. These include table sugar and the sugars found in sweets, cakes, biscuits and sweetened cereals. The sugar in these foods causes erratic fluctuations in blood sugar levels, meaning that, on consumption, you will experience a spurt of energy, followed by a dip into a low mood. Simple carbohydrates should, therefore, be avoided as much as possible.

Recommended carbohydrate consumption

I reiterate that we should all try to eat at least five portions of fruit and vegetables a day, remembering that if they are raw, they are more nutritious than those that have been cooked. Also, it is important to buy organically grown produce. Cleanly grown fruit and vegetables can now be found on our supermarket shelves and generally cost little more than intensively grown foods.

As approximately half of our calorie intake should consist of carbohydrates, the calorific values of some recommended sources are as follows:

- 28 g (1 oz) of banana gives you 22 calories;
- 28 g (1 oz) of orange, 12 calories;
- 28 g (1 oz) of apple, 17 calories;
- 28 g (1 oz) of wholemeal pasta, 35 calories;
- 28 g (1 oz) of wholemeal (also called whole grain) bread, 38 calories;
- 28 g (1 oz) of cauliflower, 3 calories;
- 28 g (1 oz) of cabbage, 4 calories.

Fats and oils

Fats (fatty acids) are the most concentrated sources of energy in our diet – just 1 g providing the body with 9 calories of energy. Foods containing good fats – omega 3 and omega 6 oils – are crucial to good health. Oils are also a natural source of vitamin E, which is an important antioxidant (see Chapter 4 for more information about antioxidants).

You will recall from earlier that there are two distinct types of fat.

- **Saturated fat** Believed to be implicated in the development of heart disease, saturated fat comes mainly from animal sources and is generally solid at room temperature. Although margarine was, for many years, believed to be a healthier choice than butter, nutritionists have now revised their opinion. This is because in the hydrogenation process used to make margarine, some of the fats are changed into trans-fatty acids, which the body metabolizes as if they were saturated fatty acids – the same as butter. Butter is a valuable source of oils and vitamin A, but should be used very sparingly. Margarine, on the other hand, is an artificial product containing many additives – even the olive oil-based ones – so should be avoided.

- **Unsaturated fat** Also called polyunsaturated or monounsaturated fat, unsaturated fat has a protective effect on the heart and other organs. Omega 3 and omega 6 oils occur naturally in oily fish (mackerel, herring, sardines, tuna and so on), nuts and seeds, and is usually liquid at room temperature. I would recommend, then, that people with CFS/ME eat oily fish at least three times a week and cold-pressed oil (olive, rapeseed, safflower and sunflower oil) daily, for dressings and in cooking. Olive oil is best suited to cooking, however, as it is damaged less by heat than other oils.

Frying

I must add that the process of frying changes the molecular structure of foods, rendering them potentially damaging to the body. If you must fry something, it is best to use a small amount of extra virgin olive oil and cook at a low temperature. A healthier alternative is to sauté in a little water or tomato juice or else grill, bake or steam. Stir-frying is good, but cook the food in a little water, drizzling on a little olive oil afterwards.

It is important to remember never to reheat used oils, for this, too, can be harmful to the body. Store your oils in a sealed container in a cool, dark place to prevent them becoming rancid.

Eggs

You're no doubt aware that eggs are high in cholesterol, which is a type of fat. However, they also contain lecithin, which is a superb biological detergent capable of breaking down fats so that they can be utilized by the body. Lecithin also prevents the accumulation of too many acid or alkaline substances in the blood and encourages the transport of nutrients through the cell walls. Eggs should be soft-boiled or poached as a hard yolk will bind the lecithin, rendering it useless as a fat detergent.

Although I have recommended that you eat two to three eggs a week, those following this diet on a vegetarian basis should eat up to five eggs a week to obtain the necessary protein.

Recommended consumption of unsaturated fat

It is estimated that most adults consume approximately 42 per cent of their total daily calories as fat – most of that being the saturated kind. However, the recommended daily intake is 20 per cent, which is 28 g

(1 oz) and gives us only 270 calories. Eating the necessary unsaturated fats will ensure reduced calorie intake and greater energy provision.

Here are the calorific values of some fat-containing foods:

- 28 g (1 oz) oil contains 130 calories;
- 28 g (1 oz) butter, 226 calories;
- 28 g (1 oz) eggs, 80 calories;
- 28 g (1 oz) oily fish, 60 calories.

Fibre (roughage)

Fibre – formerly known as roughage – is the indigestible parts of plants. It is the cellulose fibres forming the leaf webbing in green vegetables, the skins of sweetcorn and beans and the husks of wheat and corn. Fibre – a type of carbohydrate – is found in fruit, vegetables, nuts, seeds, beans, peas, lentils, wholemeal breads and cereals (wheat, oats, rye, barley, quinoa, spelt, buckwheat, corn and so on). As mentioned earlier, a high proportion of the foods recommended in the chronic fatigue healing diet contain fibre.

It is estimated that people in the West consume only 12 g (about $\frac{1}{4}$ oz) of fibre on average per day, instead of the recommended 20–30 g (1 oz). However, the latter amount was, in fact, consumed up to the time of World War II. Fibre is useful not only because of its high nutritional value, but also because it is a bulking agent, which quickly sweeps the bowel clean, ensuring that no unhealthy waste products lurk in hidden corners.

When waste products persistently linger in the bowel – which is what happens when you have a low-fibre diet – toxins are absorbed back into the bloodstream, causing eventual weakening of the immune system. Fibre has the added benefit of aiding the slow, regulated absorption of glucose into the bloodstream, as a consequence of which the individual avoids plummeting into hunger troughs and craving sugar to raise blood sugar levels. Another advantage of fibre is that the appetite is satiated on comparatively fewer calories.

Now we have a clear idea of all the elements we need to include in our diet to give our bodies what they need to be healthy. Next, we take a look at vitamins and minerals and what happens if we are not getting enough of these vital nutrients.

4

Vital Nutrients

Vitamins, minerals, essential fatty acids, amino acids and enzymes are essential to good health. They also support the repair and regeneration of the tissues and cells. However, tests have shown that people with depressed immune systems have decreased levels of vitamin C, the B complex vitamins and betacarotene, which converts to vitamin A, and vitamin E, which is a fat-soluble vitamin. In addition, even though we certainly do not go hungry today, the average Western diet is severely lacking in nutrients. For instance, we now consume less vitamin E than did a pauper in a Victorian prison. Vitamin E is vital to the prevention and treatment of all manner of diseases.

We seldom hear mention of enzymes, which are made up of vitamins and minerals, but they are not only crucial to good digestion, they also speed up the chemical reactions within our bodies. Many enzymes are provided by fresh, raw food, but are easily destroyed in cooking and processing. To obtain the right amount, I advise that you eat two to four portions of raw fruit and/or vegetables each day.

Antioxidants

Oxygen is essential to many functions within the human body, yet, like rust to a car, is also capable of seriously affecting health and longevity.

Our lungs transfer the oxygen we breathe into the bloodstream, which carries it to every cell in the body. Once inside a cell, it is involved in turning digested food into energy. However, oxygen atoms that lack an electron are also formed during this process. Called 'free radicals', these atoms charge around looking for their missing electrons, grabbing them from cell walls or from material within the cells. As a result, the unsuspecting donor cells are left damaged.

Antioxidants are the body's defence against free radicals, for they give these scavengers the electrons they need without detriment to themselves. However, when there are insufficient antioxidants present to combat the number of free radicals, the latter are able to mount a full-scale attack on the cells. If antioxidant intake continues to be low, the damage can be so severe that even vital DNA is affected. In fact, recent research has found that disease is directly influenced by the number of free radicals present in the body.

As you may have guessed, people with CFS/ME are known to be encumbered with a large supply of destructive free radicals – a situation known as 'oxidative stress' (qualified nutritionists now offer a test that determines if you are suffering from this). It is vital that sufferers consume plenty of antioxidant foods and antioxidant nutritional supplements. Many vitamins and minerals contain antioxidant properties, each type having its own working domain and mode of operation. The best sources include selenium, vitamin A, vitamin C, vitamin E, garlic, carrots, broccoli, Brazil nuts and grapeseed extract products (proanthocyanidins) – further sources are outlined later in this chapter.

Pollutants such as car exhaust fumes, ultraviolet light (leaking through the damaged ozone layer), paint and varnish fumes and so on are thought to increase the number of free radicals in our bodies, as does smoking. Although the above antioxidants, taken daily, can reduce free radical damage, smokers would be best advised to give up smoking if this is to have any appreciable effect.

Another happy outcome of consuming the recommended daily amount of antioxidants is a longer life. When bombarded with free radicals, our cells become depleted of energy – a situation that commonly leads to chronic disease. Eventually, the attacked cells die, which is detrimental to the individual. However, antioxidant-containing foods and supplements are capable of reversing any damage, allowing the cells to be far more productive.

Vitamins

Unlike proteins, carbohydrates and fats, vitamins do not provide energy or act as building materials. Their chief function is to sustain and regulate certain biochemical processes, including cellular reproduction, digestion and the metabolic rate.

Vitamins are organic food substances found only in plants and animals. Because they ensure the normal functioning of our bodies, intake must be adequate. However, due to the overfarming of land, lack of crop rotation and the refining and processing of foods, it is often difficult to acquire sufficient amounts, even from a good-quality, balanced diet. Our habit of overcooking vegetables then leads to a further loss in their nutritional value. Added to that fact, people with CFS/ME are known to suffer multiple vitamin deficiencies.

Unfortunately, a varied, whole food, organic diet is often insufficient to ensure optimum healing. It is important, therefore, that good-quality dietary supplements are taken daily. These generally come in tablet or capsule form and can be purchased from healthfood shops and specialist suppliers. They should be taken before meals to ensure maximum absorption. Look for supplements without added colourings, flavourings, preservatives, hydrogenated fats, gelatin and sugar and check their strength. Sadly, some supplements contain only minute amounts of the active ingredients. A good company will have a qualified nutritionist available to answer telephone queries and will train retailers to know about their products. Of course, they may still be biased towards their own products.

Below, I have included the recommended daily allowances (RDAs) of vitamins for people with CFS/ME. Although they are rather higher than the government's RDAs, the latter are meant only to prevent deficiency symptoms in healthy people. However, if you suffer adverse effects from taking the amounts recommended, reduce the dosage accordingly. It is wise anyway to let your doctor know before commencing vitamin and mineral supplementation.

Vitamin C (ascorbic acid)

One of the more potent antioxidants and detoxifiers, vitamin C is very much the stress vitamin and is probably the most important nutrient for the immune system. However, it is quickly used up in the body by smoking, alcohol consumption, surgery, trauma, stress, exposure to pollutants and the use of certain medicines. CFS/ME-friendly food sources are citrus fruits, strawberries, blackcurrants, tomatoes, broccoli, Brussel sprouts, cabbage, green melons, potatoes and peppers.

As this vitamin is easily destroyed by heat and overprocessing, it is recommended that vegetables be steamed for as little time as possible.

Vitamin C deficiency is characterized by bleeding gums, swollen and/or painful joints, nosebleeds, loss of appetite, muscular weakness, slow-healing wounds, easy bruising, frequent infections, anaemia and impaired digestion.

The government's recommended daily amount (RDA) is 60 mg. However, the RDA for people with CFS/ME is 1000–3000 mg, depending on the severity of symptoms.

Vitamin A (betacarotene – the precursor to retinol)

Also a powerful antioxidant, vitamin A is necessary for the growth and repair of all the body's tissues. In addition, it reduces susceptibility to infections in the nose, mouth, throat and lungs and helps to protect against pollutants. It is also very important to the immune system.

CFS/ME-friendly food sources are yellow and orange fruits and vegetables such as carrots, sweet potatoes, apricots, cantaloupe, papaya, pumpkin, melon and mango. This vitamin can also be found in dark, leafy vegetables, such as spinach, broccoli, cabbage and parsley.

Symptoms of deficiency are a susceptibility to infections, poor growth and development, rough, dry, scaly skin, loss of sense of smell and appetite, dry eyes, fatigue and defective teeth and gums.

The RDA is 3333 IU for males and 2667 IU for females. However, the RDA for those with CFS/ME is 10,000 IU. It is very important that pregnant women never take more than 10,000 IU per day as greater amounts can cause birth defects such as a cleft palate.

Vitamin E

Another major antioxidant, vitamin E helps to supply oxygen to all the organs in the body, helping to alleviate fatigue. It also nourishes the cells, protects red blood cells from toxins and aids in the maintenance of nerve and muscle function. However, as it has anti-thrombin properties, people on warfarin should consult their doctor before taking vitamin E supplements.

CFS/ME-friendly food sources are mostly oil, seed and grain derivatives. These include wheatgerm, safflower, avocados, nuts, sunflower oil and seeds, pumpkin seeds, linseeds, almonds, Brazils, cashews, pecans, whole grain cereals and breads, wheatgerm, asparagus, dried prunes and broccoli. Because rancid oils are extremely damaging to the body, oil-containing foods should be kept in an airtight container away from sunlight.

Symptoms of vitamin E deficiency are dry skin, decline in sexual vitality, abnormal fat deposits in the muscles, degenerative changes in the heart and the muscles and the onset of autoimmune disease.

The RDA is 10 mg. However, the RDA for those with CFS/ME is 200–400 mg.

B complex vitamins

The B vitamins are not only required at every stage in the creation of energy in the body, they also help to promote relaxation. Regular intakes of this vitamin are, therefore, required in the treatment of CFS/ME.

Vitamin B1 (thiamine)

This vitamin is essential for blood cell metabolism, muscle metabolism, digestion, pain inhibition and energy production.

CFS/ME-friendly food sources are oatmeal, whole wheat, brown rice, bran, wheatgerm, lentils, lean meats, free-range eggs, dried beans, sunflower seeds, peanuts and kelp. Herbs containing B1 are peppermint, slippery elm, ginseng, gotu kola.

Deficiency problems include burning and tingling in the toes and soles of the feet, depression, fatigue, muscle weakness, difficulty sleeping, irritability and loss of appetite.

The RDA is 1.5 mg for males and 1.1 mg for females. However, the RDA for those with CFS/ME is 30 mg, for both sexes.

Vitamin B2 (riboflavin)

This vitamin is necessary for cell respiration, antibody formation and the metabolizing of fats and carbohydrates. Levels of this vitamin in the body can, however, be reduced by caffeine, alcohol and some antibiotics.

CFS/ME-friendly food sources are peanuts, free-range eggs, lean meats, soya products, whole grains and leafy green vegetables.

Deficiency symptoms include insomnia, dry, cracked lips, a red, scaly nose, gritty eyes, sore lips and tongue and photophobia (light-sensitive eyes).

The RDA is 1.7 mg for males and 1.3 mg for females. However, the RDA for those with CFS/ME is 25 mg.

Vitamin B3 (niacinamide)

Due to its role in the conversion of carbohydrates into energy, this vitamin is important in treating CFS/ME. It is also involved in blood circulation and the production of several hormones (see below for details of NADH – a potent energizer derived from vitamin B3).

CFS/ME-friendly food sources are white meat, whole wheat, oily fish, avocados, nuts, peanuts, sunflower seeds, whole grains and prunes.

B3 deficiency can cause fatigue, muscle weakness, hypoglycaemia, confusion, memory loss, irritability, diarrhoea, depression, insomnia and ringing in the ears.

The RDA is 1.1 mg, but for those with CFS/ME it is 100 mg.

Vitamin B5 (pantothenic acid)
Not only is vitamin B5 crucial for the production of the anti-stress hormones, it is also vital to the release of energy from protein, carbohydrates, fats and sugars and for good health of the nervous system. In addition, this vitamin is a highly successful treatment for adrenal exhaustion, which is a common complication arising with CFS/ME (see Chapter 7 for more information on adrenal exhaustion).

Symptoms of B5 deficiency include muscle pain, dizzy spells, skin abnormalities, digestive problems, poor muscle coordination, restlessness, fatigue, depression and insomnia.

CFS/ME-friendly food sources are whole grains, soft-boiled egg yolks, fish, brewer's yeast, peanuts, walnuts, dried pears and apricots, dates and mushrooms. The RDA is 6 mg, but in CFS/ME, 250–500 mg is recommended.

Vitamin B6 (pyridoxine)
Vitamin B6 is needed for the conversion of fats and proteins into energy. It is also important for those who suffer from excessive stress.

CFS/ME-friendly food sources are bananas, whole grain bread, lean meats, eggs, dried beans, avocados, seeds, nuts, chicken, fish and liver.

Symptoms of B6 deficiency include nervousness, depression, muscle weakness, pain, headaches, irritability, stiff joints and PMS in women.

The RDA is 2 mg. The safety of vitamin B6 supplementation has been under the spotlight in recent years, but 50 mg is considered safe, even for long-term use, for those with CFS/ME.

Vitamin B12 (cobalamin)
This vitamin is crucial to protein, carbohydrate and fat metabolism, red blood cell formation and the longevity of cells. It also has the ability to strengthen the nervous system. However, many people with CFS/ME are known to have low concentrations of this vitamin in their cerebrospinal fluid, as do victims of other chronic fatigue conditions. Sufferers have reported increased energy and well-being 12–24 hours after a high-dose injection of cyanocobalamin, which is a form of vitamin B12. The effects lasted for two or three days.

Vitamin B12 deficiency is linked with abnormal immune response, poor neurological function, muscle weakness, fatigue, depression, paranoia, memory loss and headaches.

CFS/ME-friendly food sources are soft-boiled egg yolks, fish, shellfish, lean meats and poultry. As B12 is almost exclusively found in animal products, supplementation is essential for vegetarians and vegans.

The RDA is 1 mcg. However, for those with CFS/ME, it is 250 mcg, taken orally. People having injections may be given in the region of 3000 mcg on each occasion.

Vitamin P (bioflavonoids and proanthocyanidins)

Because they work with vitamin C, bioflavonoids are essential for people with CFS/ME. Natural plant bioflavonoids – such as rutin, hesperidin and quercetin – help to strengthen blood vessels and capillaries. They also help to improve the energy production process and reduce the amount of damage caused by free radicals.

Although these substances are found in virtually all plant foods, the best CFS/ME-friendly food sources are fresh fruit and vegetables, pulses, whole grains, seeds, nuts, spinach, apricots, cherries, grapes, blackberries and tea. Bioflavonoid-containing herbs and spices include paprika and rosehips. Milk thistle seed, ginkgo biloba and pycnogenol (which is obtained from the French maritime pine tree) are high in bioflavonoids and can be purchased in tablet form from healthfood shops and specialist suppliers.

There is no government RDA for bioflavonoids and proanthocyanidins. People with CFS/ME should try to consume the above foods and, if they wish, take milk thistle and ginkgo biloba supplements, closely following the dosage instructions on the container. (More about milk thistle and ginkgo biloba later.)

NADH (nicotinamide adenine dinucleotide)

Derived from vitamin B3, this coenzyme is believed by many to be the secret weapon in the war against CFS/ME. This is because it enables the body to increase adenine triphosphate (ATP) – the fuel that provides the body with energy. NADH also helps to boost the immune system by increasing the effectiveness of white blood cell function and helps to repair cellular damage. The ensuing benefits include increased energy and muscle strength, improved concentration and short-term memory, reduced pain and better sleep.

In one study[3] of 26 CFS/ME patients over 12 weeks, half the participants received Enada (a brand-named NADH supplement) during the first month while the other half received a placebo. None of the participants was told what they were taking. During the second month, no one received treatment, while in the third month, the groups were switched. The outcome was that 31 per cent of CFS/

ME sufferers reported a reduction in symptoms, while only 8 per cent of those taking the placebo did so. However, over a much longer period, 80 per cent of sufferers reported improvements in their condition.

As people with CFS/ME need a higher dosage than most, the RDA is 15–30 mg, depending on the severity of symptoms. The dosage should be reduced to 5 mg per day when symptoms improve. NADH is slowly gaining in popularity, but may not yet be available in all healthfood shops.

Biotin

This vitamin reduces stress, aids in the absorption of nutrients and is especially beneficial for those on a poor-quality diet. It aids protein, carbohydrate and fat metabolism, cell growth and energy metabolism.

CFS/ME-friendly food sources are lean meats, soft-boiled egg yolks and whole grains.

Biotin deficiency is characterized by muscle pain, fatigue, depression, nausea, anaemia, hair loss, anorexia, dermatitis and high cholesterol levels.

The RDA is 150 mcg, but for those with CFS/ME, it is 400 mcg.

Minerals

As minerals and trace elements are our most essential nutrients, the body requires small amounts of a wide range of them on a daily basis to ensure normal functioning of all its systems. Minerals are also essential to the process of waste elimination and for bringing oxygen and nutrients to the cells. They are vital for the various operations of carbohydrates, fats, vitamins, enzymes and amino acids, too.

Sadly, the use of organophosphates (weedkillers, chemical pesticides and so on) is causing minerals to rapidly disappear from our soils, as government studies have shown. Soil overuse means our food has lower levels of minerals, leading to deficiencies. This situation is made worse by prolonged stress and anxiety – another cause of low levels of minerals in the body. To compound the situation, people with CFS/ME are known to have mineral deficiencies, which leads to shortfalls in protein and vitamins. It is, therefore, important that those with CFS/ME take mineral and trace element supplements.

It is essential that the supplements you choose have a high

absorption rate for this ensures that a substantial amount is taken into the bloodstream to be used by the body. All mineral supplements are chelated (bound) to something else and what this something is determines the amount of mineral absorbed by the body. Inorganic chelates are naturally occurring mined minerals that are not easily absorbed. For example, post-menopausal women may take calcium carbonate to protect them from osteoporosis, but its absorption may be as little as 5 per cent – that's only 50 mg from a 1000-mg supplement. Oxides, sulphates and phosphates are also inorganic chelates and may not be very useful either. Organic chelates, on the other hand, can achieve up to 60 per cent absorption. Thus, while the number of milligrams you take may be smaller than for inorganic chelates, the body will absorb far greater amounts. Check the label and choose supplements with amino acid chelate, citrate, picolinate or glycinate.

Because organically chelated minerals are more expensive to produce, the cost to the consumer is greater than that of their inorganic counterparts. However, the cost is more than made up for by their far superior effects.

The following are important minerals.

Calcium

This vital mineral is the most abundant in the body, 99 per cent of it being found in the bones and teeth. It works with magnesium to ensure proper muscle contraction/relaxation and is important to the functioning of the nervous system. Calcium builds and maintains strong bones and teeth, aids the passage of nutrients into the cell walls and is essential to normal kidney function.

A deficiency of calcium is common and can be signalled by muscle cramps, tingling in the lips, fingers and feet, leg numbness, tooth decay, sensitivity to noise, depression and deterioration of the bones (osteoporosis). Too much calcium is known to be implicated in bone brittleness. However, the addition of sufficient magnesium allows the bones to have the necessary 'give' to counteract jarring and sudden impacts.

The richest sources of magnesium are also the richest sources of essential fatty acids. They include tinned sardines and salmon (including the bones), beans, nuts, seeds and whole grains. Other sources include root and leafy green vegetables, dried peas, parsley and oranges. We generally link calcium with dairy produce, but a low-dairy diet is advisable for people with CFS/ME. For that reason, a multimineral supplement should make up the shortfall.

The RDA is 800 mg, but those with CFS/ME should take 1000 mg.

Magnesium

This mineral is important for the absorption of calcium, phosphorus, potassium, vitamins C and E and the B complex vitamins. It helps to make bones less prone to breakage, and, together with calcium and vitamin C, aids the conversion of blood sugar into energy. Magnesium deficiency is as common as that of calcium, however, and, due to the precarious balance between these two associated minerals, deficiency may be caused by excessive calcium supplementation. For this reason, the ratio of calcium to magnesium intake should be approximately two to one, except where there is a deficiency of either of these minerals.

Tests have shown that many people with CFS/ME have low red blood cell magnesium levels. In fact, poor magnesium status can actually cause chronic fatigue and a susceptibility to infection. For this reason, magnesium supplementation should be higher than the recommended two to one ratio for those with CFS/ME.

The symptoms of deficiency include muscle pain and tenderness, fatigue, migraine and headaches, tremor and shakiness, poor mental function, allergies, palpitations and numbness and tingling in the fingers and toes. Magnesium levels can be lowered by consumption of caffeine and saturated fats. Acute magnesium deficiency can result from the use of diuretics, antibiotics and chemotherapy treatment. However, research has shown that magnesium supplementation produces good results in people with CFS/ME.

CFS/ME-friendly food sources include whole grains, leafy green vegetables, nuts – especially almonds and cashews – seeds, pulses, soya products, vegetables – especially broccoli and sweetcorn – and bananas and apricots.

The RDA is 270 mg. However, for those with CFS/ME, 600–1200 mg is advised.

Manganese

Manganese is an important antioxidant for people with CFS/ME as it helps the body to create energy from glucose. It also aids in the normalization of the central nervous system, activates enzymes known to be helpful in the digestion and utilization of foods and plays a key role in the breakdown of fats and cholesterol.

CFS/ME-friendly food sources are leafy green vegetables, whole grains, nuts, seeds and tea. Deficiency symptoms include digestive problems, dizziness, paralysis and convulsions.

The RDA for CFS/ME is 10 mg.

Zinc

Another powerful antioxidant, zinc is involved in a wide range of metabolic activities, including digestion, protein synthesis and insulin production. It is also required for the healthy functioning of the immune system and the development and maintenance of the reproductive organs. This mineral is generally low in Western foods, but people with CFS/ME are often particularly deficient. Vegetarian diets can easily have shortfalls of zinc, too, because the high grain content binds to this mineral, rendering it useless. It should be accompanied by copper in a ratio of 10–15 mg of zinc to 1 mg of copper, to prevent a possible copper imbalance.

Deficiency symptoms include white spots on the fingernails, stretch marks, fatigue, decreased alertness and a susceptibility to infections.

CFS/ME-friendly food sources are liquorice, seafood, lean meats, eggs, liver, wheatgerm, pumpkin seeds, sunflower seeds and ginseng.

The RDA is 9.5 mg, but people with CFS/ME require 15 mg daily.

Selenium

A major antioxidant, this mineral protects the cells from the toxic effects of free radicals and, in so doing, boosts the immune system. By means of oxidation, selenium slows down the ageing and hardening of tissues, thus preserving tissue elasticity. It also aids DNA repair, triggers thyroid hormone activation and helps to protect against cancer.

Selenium deficiency symptoms include frequent infections, premature ageing, poor detoxification, cataracts, cancerous changes, loose skin, dandruff and heart disease.

CFS/ME-friendly food sources are tuna, salmon, shrimps, garlic, tomatoes, sunflower seeds, Brazil nuts and wheat breads.

The RDA is 75 mcg, but people with CFS/ME require 100 mcg.

Potassium

This mineral works with sodium to regulate the functioning of the heart and muscles. It also ensures the correct acid/alkaline balance, normal transmission of nerve impulses, stability of internal cell structure and stimulation of the kidneys to eliminate toxic body waste.

Deficiency symptoms include intense thirst, bloating, dizziness, low blood pressure, poor reflexes, muscle twitches, acute muscle weakness, nervous disorders, erratic and/or rapid heartbeats, insomnia, fatigue and high cholesterol levels.

CFS/ME-friendly food sources are bananas, lean meats, avocados, tomato juice, fruit and vegetable juices, nuts, salad vegetables, potatoes, oranges and dried fruits.

The RDA is 3500 mg. However, the RDA for those with CFS/ME is 5000 mg.

Chromium

Chromium is part of what is known as the 'glucose tolerance factor', which works with the B vitamins and magnesium to metabolize sugar and stabilize blood sugar levels. As chromium is lost in the urine whenever sugar is consumed, a high intake of sugar can lead to chromium deficiency. The latter is characterized by weight loss, glucose intolerance, tiredness, diabetes and heart disease.

CFS/ME-friendly food sources are brewer's yeast, liver, whole grains, mushrooms and low-fat organic cheese.

The RDA for CFS/ME is 200 mcg.

A note about dosages

It is important to note that, in most instances, the RDAs of vitamin and mineral supplements set by the UK Department of Health are only intended to prevent common diseases associated with a severe deficiency, not promote the optimal functioning and protection of bodily systems. RDAs, therefore, are the very minimum requirement for good health. For example, the RDA for vitamin E is 10 mg, but research has shown that the level offering protection to the heart is in excess of 67 mg daily. Of course, this amount includes vitamin E obtained from food sources.

Other useful supplements

Malic acid

This supplement plays a vital role in the operation of the important malic acid shuttle service, which delivers important nutrients to the cells. Malic acid enters the cycle at the most efficient site and is then converted into usable energy. It is particularly effective when combined with magnesium. Some supplement manufacturers now offer magnesium malate, which combines the two.

CFS/ME-friendly food sources are all fruits, but apples have by far the highest content. The RDA for those with CFS/ME is 200 mg.

Co-enzyme Q10

Also known as CoQ10, this enzyme is an important aid to people with CFS/ME as it helps to increase energy and alleviate fatigue. A powerful antioxidant, it works by aiding the transfer of oxygen and energy between components of the cells and between the blood and tissues. It also benefits the immune system, reduces allergic response and improves concentration and short-term memory.

CFS/ME-friendly food sources are peanuts, mackerel, nuts, chicken, whole grains, wild salmon, sardines and spinach. CoQ10 can be purchased in capsule form from healthfood shops and specialist supplement suppliers. The RDA for people with CFS/ME is 100 mg.

Boron

This trace element is thought to be involved in bone mineralization and is important to maintaining good muscular health. Because people with CFS/ME may be inactive for long periods, it is also useful for reducing calcium loss, particularly in post-menopausal women. In countries where high levels of boron remain in the soil, it has been found that there are the lowest incidences of arthritis.

Deficiency symptoms are thought to include osteoporosis and menopausal symptoms in women.

CFS/ME-friendly food sources are apples, pears, prunes, seeds, raisins, tomatoes and cauliflower.

The RDA for CFS/ME is 3 mg.

Ginkgo biloba

This herbal antioxidant is useful for improving blood circulation. As a result, cognitive function (concentration, memory and so on) is improved, as is energy production. In two trials undertaken in the 1990s, volunteers were given ginkgo biloba daily. The first trial[4] showed that their short-term memories had improved significantly and, in the second,[5] the volunteers displayed even sharper reactions and recall, as well as improved brain function – all of which were judged to be due to their improved circulation. Ginkgo biloba is, therefore, considered very useful in the treatment of CFS/ME.

This herb can be purchased in capsule form from healthfood

shops, some pharmacies and larger supermarkets and the dosage instructions on the packaging should be followed. As people taking prescription medication – warfarin and aspirin – can react adversely to this supplement, please consult your doctor before use.

Oil of evening primrose

This essential fatty acid of the omega 6 family is extracted from the seed of the evening primrose plant. It contains gamma linolenic acid (GLA), which, in turn, is a vital link in prostaglandin manufacture. (Prostaglandins are hormone-like substances involved in reducing inflammation in the body.)

However, conversion of linolenic acid (omega 6) to GLA can be slowed down by foods rich in saturated fat, alcohol, excessive sugar, zinc deficiency, stress and ageing. When omega 6 conversion to GLA is inefficient, supplementation is highly recommended. Oil of evening primrose is often taken by women prior to menstruation to help maintain GLA levels. Because it aids hormone balance, it is also recommended for people with CFS/ME.

The RDA is 500–1000 mg.

Echinacea

One of the most researched of all herbs, echinacea has broad antibiotic properties, much like penicillin. Besides acting as a stimulant to the immune system, aiding the destruction of germs, it is also capable of strengthening cell defences. As an antiviral agent, echinacea may be used by people with CFS/ME at first indications of a cold or flu to lessen the severity of the illness. Some sufferers report a reduction in all symptoms as a result of taking this herb regularly. However, it is possible that people with overactive immune systems (generally those with more severe CFS/ME symptoms) may suffer adverse effects.

Alcohol-free tinctures are now available in most healthfood shops. Alternatively, dry echinacea root – also available in healthfood shops – can be infused to make tea.

Rhodiola rosea

This powerful Russian nutrient belongs to the family of adaptogenic herbs – those that encourage the body to adapt to stress. Research has shown that rhodiola rosea has a protective effect on the immune system, boosts sexual function, helps to raise energy levels, increases resistance to disease and aids detoxification. It also has revitalizing properties and helps to stabilize mood swings.

Most healthfood shops now stock this stress-busting adaptogen, as do specialist supplement manufacturers (see the Useful Addresses section at the back of this book for further details). The RDA for CFS/ME is 180 mg.

Ashwagandha

Also an adaptogenic herb, ashwagandha – sometimes called Indian ginseng – is an important tonic, containing a broad range of important healing powers rare in the plant kingdom. Not only is it good for restoring energy in people with chronic fatigue, it has also been shown in research to help rejuvenate the nervous system, enhance memory and concentration and ease insomnia and stress.

In one double-blind study (where neither the researchers nor those taking part know who is receiving the medicine and who is receiving an inert substitute, called a placebo),[6] 101 healthy middle-aged men took either ashwagandha or a placebo for one year. As a result, the indications of ageing – such as greying hair and low calcium levels – were found to be significantly improved in those taking ashwagandha. Also, 70 per cent of this section also reported increased libido and sexual function.

Ashwagandha can be found in most healthfood shops and is available from specialist supplement manufacturers. The RDA for CFS/ME is 750 mg.

Siberian ginseng

The many benefits of Siberian ginseng – the most well known of the adaptogenic herbs – include increased physical endurance under stress, protection against infection, protection against excessive cold and heat, improved hormone activity and better sexual function. In a recent study, those taking Siberian ginseng showed significant improvements in immune system function. It is now often given to Russian combat troops when embarking on active manoeuvres.

This very safe herb is available from most healthfood shops and specialist supplement manufacturers. The RDA is 2–4 g for the dried root, 10–20 ml for the tincture, 2–4 ml for the fluid extract and 100–200 mg for the solid extract. People with CFS/ME should take double these amounts.

Guidance on taking supplements

As vitamins A, C and E (known as the ACE vitamins), together with CoQ10, selenium, zinc and manganese, work as fine antioxidants, I strongly recommend that they form your first line of defence. These substances may be purchased together in a single, high-potency antioxidant supplement from specialist suppliers and are sold under various brand names (see the Useful Addresses section for details of recommended antioxidant suppliers). The multiantioxidant supplement will often also contain other important nutrients. Alternatively, the constituents may be bought separately, but generally at a higher overall price. Trials have shown that the above-mentioned combination of antioxidants should be taken for a period of one month before commencing further radical supplementation. However, B complex supplementation and evening primrose oil could be started after two weeks.

During month two, I suggest that you begin taking one of the adaptogenic herbs – rhodiola rosea, Siberian ginseng and ashwagandha help to normalize and regulate the various systems within the body, promoting health and wellbeing, and so are very useful in treating CFS/ME. You could then start magnesium and malic acid supplementation, which work together to reduce fatigue, pain and low muscle stamina. However, in the main, these two constituents can only be bought separately (see the Useful Addresses section for details of suppliers who sell a combination supplement called magnesium malate).

A multimineral and trace element supplement containing calcium, magnesium, manganese, zinc, boron, potassium and chromium should also be taken after a further two weeks. Most people find that a liquid formulation gives greater absorption than does the tablet form (see the Useful addresses section for suppliers).

During month three, you may wish to begin taking ginkgo biloba and CoQ10, which work to improve brain function and energy production. However, check that these nutrients are not already included in your antioxidant preparation. Echinacea – the immune system stimulant – could be sampled for reaction in month four – most sufferers should be able to tolerate it.

I can almost hear some of you protesting about the expense at this point. Unfortunately, because of the many deficiencies in CFS/ME, supplementation is very important. Apart from following the recommended diet, there is, to date, no better way to significantly reduce symptoms. By following the diet alone, you should, in time, see a noticeable difference in your health, but, by incorporating the recommended supplements as well, you will give your body an even greater chance of healing. Having said that, please remember that to take only one or two types of supplements is better than none at all. The antioxidant preparation is of prime importance, as is the magnesium malate, closely followed by the liquid mineral and trace element formulation.

As we are all very different, I would advise that you test the effects of each supplement to assess the required dosage, maybe even commencing each type of supplement separately to judge its effects more accurately. You may actually require a higher or lower dose than initially supposed. However, you should reduce a high dose after a maximum of eight to ten months as an oversupply may create its own imbalance. I must add that if you still feel no real benefit after sampling a higher dose of a particular supplement for six to eight weeks, you should discontinue its use.

If you are still unsure about which supplements to take, I suggest that you consult a nutritionist. They will not only assess your particular requirements and give clear dosage instructions, but also guide you through the diet.

It is important to note that when a person begins taking a course of supplements, the body may immediately start to detoxify, releasing stored toxins and debris into the bloodstream. This may cause adverse reactions, such as headaches and lethargy, for a day or so, until the loosened toxins are eliminated from the body. Try not to be overly concerned about this. It is a sure sign that you are on the way to better health.

Unfortunately, intolerances to supplements used repeatedly can occur, just as they can do to foods. For this reason, it is important to continue to closely monitor your reactions. Changing your supplement brands every now and again should avoid this risk.

5
Foods to Avoid

Unfortunately, there are many foods that lead to food allergies/intolerances and irritable bowel syndrome (IBS) and, ultimately, suppress the immune system. Although some of these foods have been mentioned previously, I think we should look at them in further detail here.

Stimulants

You may be interested to know that experts believe one of the main reasons we crave stimulants such as alcohol, caffeine, cigarettes and products containing white refined sugar is high levels of stress. When we are overworked, anxious or suffering from stress, our bodies demand a boost of energy, a 'lift'. However, the lift we obtain from such stimulants is short-lived, but the damage to our bodies can affect us in the long term.

Cutting out stimulants can significantly raise energy levels, reduce anxiety and greatly improve cell health. If you find you are unable to completely eliminate stimulants from your diet, however, reduce them as much as possible – it will make a difference. Allowing yourself an occasional treat may make this diet easier to adhere to – so long as the treats don't then become routine! Obviously smoking does not count. If you manage to cut out smoking, an occasional cigarette will risk undoing all your hard work.

Caffeine
Caffeine products – which include coffee, tea, cocoa, cola drinks and chocolate – cause stress to the adrenal glands. They are also toxic to the liver and can reduce the body's ability to absorb vitamins and minerals. Caffeine, being closely related to cocaine, morphine, strychnine and nicotine, which are all nerve poisons, is detrimental to the nervous system, too. Consumed regularly in fairly large quantities, it is likely to give rise to chronic anxiety, the symptoms of which are agitation, palpitations, headaches, indigestion, panic, insomnia and hyperventilation. My best advice is to remove caffeine products from your diet.

The addictiveness of caffeine makes reducing your consumption of it far from easy, however, and withdrawal symptoms can take the form of splitting headaches, fatigue, depression, poor concentration and muscle pains. It's no wonder people can feel terrible until they have had their first dose of caffeine in the morning and can't seem to function properly without regular doses throughout the day! Fortunately, caffeine is quickly 'washed out' of the system and it is possible to minimize withdrawal symptoms by reducing intakes over several weeks.

A problem for many is finding an acceptable alternative. Coffee, tea, cocoa and cola drinks can be replaced by fruit and vegetable juices, herbal teas. Green tea is very good, as is rooibosch (redbush) tea and they are both low in tannin and high in antioxidants. A variety of grain coffee substitutes may also be purchased from healthfood shops. As many decaffeinated products are processed with the use of chemicals, unfortunately they are not a good substitute.

Carob, which is similar to the cocoa bean, is a healthy, caffeine-free alternative to cocoa and chocolate. It contains less fat and is naturally sweet, unlike the cocoa bean, which is bitter and needs sweetening. Most people find carob bars an enjoyable replacement for chocolate bars and other confectionery. It is also available in powder form for use in baking and drinks.

Alcohol

Many CFS/ME sufferers cannot tolerate alcohol, some saying it causes their blood to run like acid through their veins. Furthermore, it appears that the more some sufferers drink, the more severe their symptoms become. These responses point to poor liver function, which can actually be tested for.

Unfortunately, alcohol – a toxin – acts on the central nervous system, which is often highly sensitized in those with CFS/ME anyway. As herbal tinctures usually contain small amounts of alcohol, they too will not be tolerated by those who are especially sensitive to it.

Because antioxidants are required to mop up the damaging free radicals stimulated by the liver's alcohol detoxification process, alcohol consumption can deplete antioxidant supplies. Even more damaging is the fact that pesticides, colourants and other harmful additives are generally involved in modern-day alcohol production, exerting further strain on the liver. For these reasons, even those with CFS/ME who do not have an immediate adverse reaction to alcohol would be best advised to avoid it as it may cause problems later and certainly will not have any beneficial effects in the meantime.

Sugar

Refined white sugar has been dubbed one of the greatest health hazards in the Western world. Sugar tastes good, but it has no nutritional value and depletes our bodies of chromium and the B vitamins – all of which are necessary for sugar metabolism. Furthermore, it fills us up in place of the foods our bodies need. Sugar is added to almost all processed and preprepared foods and provides us with an instant 'lift', but to the detriment of our long-term health.

Researchers have found that many people with CFS/ME crave sugar and this appears to be because carbohydrates can be poorly metabolized, causing insufficient glucose to be manufactured by the body. When those with CFS/ME eat sugar products several times a day, blood sugar levels continuously rise and plummet, resulting, in time, in mental and physical exhaustion. Only the unrefined sugars present naturally in fruit – that is, sugar that has not undergone processing – will not cause blood sugar levels to rise and trough so sharply. I strongly recommend, therefore, that refined white sugar be removed from your diet.

If you must sweeten your food, alternatives to refined white sugar include raw honey, barley malt and fruit juice sweetener. Muscovado and demerara sugar (also called brown sugar) are formed during the early stages of the sugar-refining process and so contain far more nutrients than refined white sugar. These sugars may all be used in cooking and baking. Try to avoid artificial sweeteners, however, as they perpetuate a sweet tooth and are dubious in terms of safety.

Aspartame

Aspartame – the widely used artificial sweetener – is surrounded by controversy. When given to test monkeys, it proved harmless, but this is now believed to be due to the highly nutritious, antioxidant-rich foods consumed by these animals. Experts now conclude that aspartame is harmless to those on antioxidant-rich diets, but may cause serious problems in people who are not.

I have read several articles about the unwelcome side-effects of aspartame and have decided that perhaps people with immune system/central nervous system disorders should err on the side of caution and avoid it. It is particularly interesting that 'aspartame poisoning' is said to produce many of the symptoms and conditions occurring in those with CFS/ME. These include muscle and joint pain, depression, anxiety, fatigue and weakness, headaches, sleep problems, dizziness, diarrhoea, tinnitus, mood swings, blurred vision and short-term memory loss. Furthermore, there is increasing evidence that it can cause serious metabolic problems in CFS/ME.

Nancy Markle – an expert on multiple sclerosis – stated at a World Environment Conference that aspartame can be dangerous to diabetics, multiple sclerosis patients and people with Parkinson's disease. Neurosurgeon Dr Russell Blakelock states in his book *Excitotoxins: The Taste that Kills* (Health Press Books, 1996) that the ingredients of aspartame can overstimulate the neurons of the brain, giving rise to dangerous symptoms. Furthermore, Dr H. J. Roberts, a diabetic specialist, has written in his book *Defense Against Alzheimer's Disease* (Sunshine Sentinel Press Inc., 1995) that aspartame poisoning is escalating Alzheimer's disease.

In an article, Nancy Markle writes that there were speakers and ambassadors from different nations at the World Environment Conference who promised to help spread the word. She added that there is actually no reason to use aspartame and that it is not, in effect, a diet product. The congressional record says, 'It [aspartame] causes a craving for carbohydrates and will cause weight gain.' One doctor revealed that when he got people off aspartame, their average weight loss was 8.5 kg (19 lbs) per person.

I would advise, therefore, that if the label says 'sugar-free' or 'diet', check the list of ingredients. Please be aware, too, that NutraSweet and Equal are brand names for aspartame.

Food additives

The majority of the foods on our supermarket shelves have undergone some degree of refinement or chemical alteration that may give rise to sensitivity reactions. These reactions include stomach upsets, inflammation, itching, headaches, pain, insomnia, depression and hyperactivity. Food additives are now believed to contribute to the onset of CFS/ME, as well as relapses.

The food additives to which people with CFS/ME are most sensitive are the following.

- **MSG** Monosodium glutamate is now the most commonly used flavour-enhancer. As manufacturers are not required to call it MSG on the label, it is often disguised as yeast food, hydrolyzed yeast, autolyzed yeast, yeast extract, sodium caseinate, natural flavouring, vegetable protein, hydrolyzed protein, other spices and natural chicken or turkey flavouring. This product is particularly detrimental to CFS/ME sufferers as it can trigger neurological allergy symptoms, such as sneezing, itching, hives, headaches, bloating, upset stomach, excessive thirst, restlessness, chest pain, joint pain and severe depression.

- **Artificial colourings** Derived from petroleum, artificial colourings contain toxic compounds that have been linked to cancer, bladder polyps, adrenal exhaustion, kidney lesions and impaired thyroid function.
- **BHA** A widely used preservative, butylated hydroxyanisole is added to baked goods, breakfast cereals, potatoes, pastry mixes, dry mixes for desserts, chewing gum, sweets, ice cream and other foods. BHA can adversely affect liver and kidney function and has been associated with behavioural problems in children.
- **BHT** Butylated hydroxytoluene is used to preserve pork sausages and freeze-dried meats. It is also added to chewing gum. Health risks from this product include allergic reactions and liver damage.
- **Sorbate** A preservative and fungus preventative, sorbate can be found in drinks, baked goods, pie fillings, artificially sweetened jellies, preserves, deli salads and fresh fruit cocktails. It is known to be detrimental to overall health.
- **Sulfites** Used in the bleaching and preserving of certain foods, this substance prevents the discoloration of light-coloured fruit and vegetables, enabling them to look fresh for longer. Sulfites are often found in beer, lager, wine and sliced fruit. They may also be present in packaged wine vinegar, gravies, avocado dip, sauces, potatoes and lemon juice. As with other food additives, sulfites are toxic substances and are particularly harmful to people with CFS/ME.
- **Aspartame** As stated earlier, aspartame has been linked with problems in many of the systems in the body. It is often found in foods described as 'low-sugar', 'sugar-free' or 'diet'. Equal and NutraSweet are brand names for aspartame.

Refined white flours

Refined wheat flour is generally known to us as plain or self-raising flour, but can also be called bread flour, pastry flour or all-purpose flour. In this instance, 'refined' means that the husks and germ of the wheat grain have been taken out and the remaining powder bleached. The result of these processes is that most of the nutritional value is removed, including vitamins, minerals, protein and the fibre. Only carbohydrates, calories and a little protein remain.

Fortified flours have, as the name implies, had some of their nutrients added. However, vitamins B6 and E and folacin are not. Also, of the nine minerals initially removed, only three – iron, calcium and phosphorus – are added, but in forms that are not easily absorbed by the body. All in all, refined flours have little nutritional value.

Healthy flours include wholemeal, spelt, quinoa, oat, maize, brown rice, rye, barley and potato, all of which are high in nutrients. Buckwheat, although not actually a grain, also makes a delicious alternative and, as with millet and rice, is free of gluten – a common allergen. Because wheatgerm is high in the B vitamins that are so important to people with CFS/ME, it is highly recommended. Granary bread, to which crushed wheat and rye grains have been added, makes a pleasant alternative. Remember that organically produced flours are best.

A word of warning – please ensure that your 'wholemeal' loaf of bread really is wholemeal and not dyed white or a mix of flours. I'm afraid 'brown' tells you nothing and is normally not much better than white bread. Bread mixes that are nutritious and easy to prepare can be purchased in healthfood shops.

People with a wheat allergy should obviously avoid this grain.

Salt

Although our bodies need the sodium we obtain from salt, high intakes of it can be harmful in many ways. High blood pressure and heart disease are just two conditions that are linked to high salt consumption.

Salt is added to virtually all processed foods as a preservative, due to its ability to inhibit the growth of harmful micro-organisms. Large amounts are also added to most breakfast cereals, except for shredded wheat products. I would recommend, therefore, that you either leave salt out of cooking altogether or use a very small amount of sea salt or rock salt. Also, avoid sprinkling any type of salt over your meals. Gradually reducing salt intake is the best way to retrain your palate.

People in hot climates and who sweat a lot should ensure that lost salt is always replaced, however, as sweating causes sodium levels to drop.

Junk food

Junk food – as its name implies – contains many ingredients that are detrimental to health. They include sugar, salt, white refined flour, saturated fat and chemical additives. Furthermore, this type of food has little nutritional value and a great deal of energy is required to digest, absorb and eliminate it.

In CFS/ME, the body is unable to find sufficient energy to complete the digestive process efficiently, as a result of which toxins and debris are stored in the body. Unfortunately, toxic buildup affects every part of the body, from the neurons of the brain to the arteries and vital organs.

6
The Detoxification Programme

It is estimated that many people carry kilos of toxic byproducts and waste in their organs and tissues, accumulated over many years. As those with CFS/ME are badly affected by 'toxic overload' (see Chapter 7 for more details), detoxification is a giant leap towards better health. Detoxification works by giving the digestive system a well-earned rest, which allows the body to focus on pulling toxic byproducts and waste from the cells into the bloodstream to be dealt with by the liver and kidneys. These organs of detoxification then work to eliminate the toxins from the body.

Detoxification is triggered by the consumption of cleansing fuel, in the form of fruit, vegetables, juices and water – all of which require minimal digestion. The energy saved is then used to eliminate toxins and debris. Requiring only slightly more digestion, whole grains and cereals, oils, nuts, seeds, herbs and spices are also useful to detoxification. As with fruit and vegetables, they are a source of vital nutrients, too.

I hardly need say that cutting down on foods we enjoy can be incredibly difficult, but cravings for these foods really can disappear, given a little time and determination. It may help to know that the people who follow this diet generally admit to finding it enjoyable after the first couple of months. Don't despair if you are unable to follow it to the letter, however, as any improvement in your diet will benefit your health, to some degree at least. Remember, studies have shown that it takes only 28 days for a food to become a habit.

The detoxification superfoods

The 21-day programme relies on the following foods, which are all powerful aids to detoxification.

Fruit

Because fruit is high in fibre and water, it is a perfect internal cleanser. The fibre binds with toxins and the water helps to flush them out. The pectin content of fruit is also useful as it binds with certain heavy metals, helping to carry them from the body.

Try to make fruit a staple of your detoxification programme, as it

49

is packed with important vitamins, minerals, amino acids and enzymes. Just to reiterate, organic fruit is best.

- **Lemons** As lemons stimulate the organs of detoxification, try to start your day with a glass of hot water with freshly squeezed lemon juice. This fruit is high in vitamin C and has cleansing and antiseptic properties.
- **Apples** The malic acid in apples is important to the release of energy. Apples also boost digestion and aid the removal of impurities from the liver. Their high fibre and pectin content assists in the elimination of toxins, helping to purify the system. Apples are rich in vitamin C, betacarotene and tartaric acid, too.
- **Oranges** Containing powerful antioxidant properties, oranges help to protect the cells. They are high in vitamin C, calcium and other nutrients.
- **Grapefruit** This fruit is rich in vitamin C, betacarotene, calcium, phosphorus and potassium.
- **Pears** Pears contain vitamin C, fibre, potassium and pectin.
- **Grapes** Not only are grapes one of the finest detoxifiers, they are also beneficial for disorders of the liver, kidneys, digestion and skin. It is vital that you buy organic grapes, though, as other ones are sprayed liberally with pesticides.
- **Bananas** Containing fibre, vitamins and potassium, bananas provide plenty of energy. This makes them a useful aid to detoxification.
- **Melons** Melons are beneficial as they contain vitamin C and betacarotene.
- **Pineapples** Possessing anti-inflammatory and antibacterial properties, pineapples also assist in the digestion of protein. They are rich in vitamin C, betacarotene, folic acid and essential minerals, too.
- **Cherries** Containing C and B vitamins and potassium, cherries aid the removal of toxins from the liver, kidneys, and digestive system. The darker the cherry, the more effective it will be.
- **Mangos** Rich in vitamin C, betacarotene and potassium, mangos are believed to cleanse the blood and benefit the kidneys.

Dried fruit also aids detoxification and is a good source of nutrients.

Raw fruit and vegetable juices
Juices derived from fresh fruit and vegetables possess remarkable healing properties, especially as part of a cleansing diet. Not only are they very easy to digest, but they also help to speed up the

metabolism, raise energy levels and stimulate detoxification. Their visible benefits include healthier-looking nails and hair.

It is important, therefore, that you try to make organically produced fruit and vegetable juices central to your programme. Juicers are inexpensive to buy and ideal for making a quick, nutritious drink. Liquidizers and blenders are great, too, for the same reason. (See Part Two for drink recipes, and the Useful Addresses section at the back of this book for details of a distributor of organic vegetable juices.)

Vegetables

Like fruit, vegetables should be a mainstay of a detoxification programme. They are full of vitamins, minerals, bioflavonoids and plant nutrients (phytochemicals). Eat raw if possible – grated carrot with salad, chopped cabbage, carrot and onion in a home-made coleslaw and celery, cauliflower, peppers and spring onions in a French dressing, for example.

When making hot meals, try to get used to eating your vegetables as lightly cooked as possible. They are more nutritious this way. Remember, too, that organic vegetables are best.

The benefits of vegetables are as follows.

- **Carrots** Excellent aids to detoxification, carrots cleanse, nourish and stimulate the whole body – particularly the kidneys, liver and digestive system. Fresh carrot juice is especially beneficial.
- **Onions, garlic and leeks** These vegetables contain fine antiviral and antibacterial nutrients and are said to cleanse the whole system. Garlic is particularly useful as it has anti-inflammatory properties and is an immune system booster. During detoxification, try to eat two cloves of raw garlic a day or take garlic supplements.
- **Broccoli, cabbage, cauliflower, Brussel sprouts and watercress** Members of the cruciferous family, these vegetables contain many nutrients that help to stimulate the liver and activate the body's enzyme defences. They therefore play a vital role in fighting disease.
- **Spinach** This leafy vegetable is rich in betacarotene, vitamin C and many more important antioxidant nutrients, making it an excellent aid to detoxification.
- **Tomatoes** Also containing many vital nutrients, tomatoes are thought to stimulate the liver and aid the removal of toxins. Vine-ripened tomatoes are best.

- **Celery** This vegetable is useful during detoxification as it can aid the removal of excess fluid from the body.
- **Cucumber** Like celery, cucumber can act as a mild diuretic. Although it has little nutritional content, it helps to improve kidney function, aids digestion and relaxes the system.
- **Beetroot** This vegetable contains potassium, sodium, iron and manganese, making it an excellent liver, kidney and gall bladder cleanser. Raw beetroot and beetroot juice work as good general tonics and are especially useful during detoxification.
- **Lettuce** Containing vitamin C, betacarotene, folate and iron, lettuce has calming, sedative properties. The darker the leaf, the more nutritious it is.

Grains

Whole grains and cereals, such as brown rice, couscous, millet, barley, oats, rye, maize, spelt and quinoa, are excellent sources of protein, complex carbohydrates, fibre, vitamins and minerals. Their starch content is absorbed quite slowly, keeping blood sugar levels steady, which is important during detoxification. However, because wheat is a common allergen that can irritate the digestive system and block the absorption of some nutrients, it should be avoided for the duration of the detoxification programme.

Pulses

The high fibre content of beans and pulses, such as lentils, soya beans, chickpeas and dried peas, makes them a vital part of a cleansing diet. They are also high in protein and other vitamins and minerals.

If you are unable to find organic beans that are canned in water, dried beans are a good alternative. However, most dried beans require soaking for at least eight hours prior to cooking. The preparation instructions should then be carefully followed, especially for red kidney beans as they can be harmful if not cooked properly.

The traditional preparation of tofu from soya beans allows nearly all the nutritious substances to be preserved. It has a subtle flavour that conveniently adapts to all types of cooking, both sweet and savoury. Tofu is also very easy to digest. (See the Useful Addresses section for details of a supplier of tofu made from organic soya and spring water.)

Although tempeh – a soya superfood – was developed in Indonesia 2000 years ago, it has only recently appeared on our supermarket shelves. Containing many important nutrients, it is a fermented product that is inoculated with healthy bacteria, which gives it a chewy, meaty texture. It takes very little preparation and cooking time and has a nutty, mushroom-like taste (see the Further Reading section for details of an excellent soya cookbook).

Nuts and seeds

Excellent sources of nutrients and omega 6 oils, nuts and seeds support the immune system during detoxification. Their other benefits include reduced risk of heart disease and certain cancers. They also improve the skin, hair and nails. A wide range of nuts should be consumed, but in moderation, as their fat content is high. Salted and coated nuts should be avoided.

Sea vegetables

Sea vegetables contain a wealth of highly nutritious vitamins and minerals, including those that are not normally obtained from other sources. Foods such as dulse, laver, nori, kelp, kombu, wakame, mekabu, hijiki, arame, agar agar and carrageen may taste a little strange at first, but most people find them delicious after the third or fourth meal. Useful ingredients in soups, salads, dressings and stocks, they are particularly beneficial during detoxification as they bind to certain heavy metals prior to eliminating them from the body (see the Further Reading section at the back of this book for details of an excellent book on the subject).

Oils and vinegars

Although unsaturated oils (fats) – those that are liquid at room temperature – are an important part of a detoxification programme, saturated fats – those that are solid at room temperature – should be avoided. Extra virgin olive oil and cold-pressed oils, such as safflower, sunflower and rapeseed, provide essential fatty acids as well as vitamin E. You may wish to try speciality oils such as almond, walnut, sesame, hemp and hazelnut.

Organic apple cider vinegar is a good source of alkaline minerals that help to rid the body of acid (people with chronic illnesses generally have overly acidic bodily tissues). Apple cider vinegar is an excellent aid to detoxification as it stimulates digestion and carries many health-giving properties. Other vinegars are not recommended as they contain acetic acid, which hinders digestion.

Spices

Many spices have a cleansing, antiseptic effect on the body. Fresh root ginger is a powerful healing spice, as are cardamom, cinnamon, cayenne, turmeric, nutmeg and fenugreek.

Sprouting

When foods are sprouted, dormant enzymes spring into action, providing more nutrients per gram than any other natural food. Eating a mixture of different sprouts is even capable of keeping you alive if you exclude all other foods, although this is not recommended! Sprouted foods are also very inexpensive. For this reason, you may wish to try them.

Fresh seeds, beans and grains will sprout when rinsed and then placed in pure water in a plastic bowl or polythene bag. The container should be sealed and placed in an airing cupboard or by a radiator for three to four days, ensuring that you change the water twice a day. A dose of light and sunshine will make them ready for eating. Be aware, though, that seed potatoes and tomatoes should not be sprouted as they belong to the deadly nightshade family. Kidney bean sprouts are poisonous, too. (See the Useful Addresses section at the back of this book for details of a book devoted to the art of sprouting.)

Organic live yogurt

Many people with CFS/ME are prone to suffering from chronic candida (yeast) infection. The infection then exacerbates the CFS/ME symptoms and creates other symptoms of its own. However, organic natural live yogurt contains beneficial bacteria that help to combat an overgrowth of candida within the gut. It is especially helpful when sugar and yeasts are removed from the diet (see Chapter 7 for more information on candida infections). Try to eat a helping of natural live yogurt every day during detoxification.

Herbs

Long valued for their therapeutic qualities, herbs can be helpful for people with CFS/ME. Fresh and dried herbs can be used in tea infusions or cooking, and herbal remedies come in the form of tinctures or tablets to take orally or as poultices for topical application. Because people with CFS/ME rarely benefit from a mixture of herbs, they are best taken singly.

Teas should be prepared by steeping the leaves in 300 ml ($\frac{1}{2}$ pint) of boiling water for 10 to 15 minutes. If the bark or root is used, place the water in the pan and boil for 15 minutes. Drink no more than two cups of a herbal tea per day for no more than two weeks. The majority of herbal tinctures are prepared with the use of alcohol.

However, if you suffer from alcohol sensitivity, some alcohol-free tinctures are now being produced.

The herbs that offer most benefit for people with CFS/ME in terms of detoxification include astragalus, gotu kola, goldenseal, echinacea and milk thistle. Because these herbs have powerful properties, it is important to follow the label dosage instructions and closely monitor your reactions. Too much of a particular herb may aggravate your symptoms.

Avoiding meat and dairy products

Animal protein foods, such as meat and dairy products, should be avoided during detoxification as they use a great deal of energy in their digestion and elimination. In addition, dairy products form mucus, which can even lurk in the bowel, where it slows the transport of waste material, hampering the elimination of toxins and debris. As animals are generally reared with the use of hormones, antibiotics and pesticides, any meat and dairy products you do eat should be organic. Alternatives include soya, rice and goats' milk and cheese, beans, pulses and soya products.

Weight matters

Because those with CFS/ME are comparatively inactive because of the symptoms, some may become overweight. Conditions related to excess weight include high blood pressure, heart disease, diabetes, chronic anxiety and depression. Crash diets and those that limit certain foods may result in substantial weight loss in the early weeks, but the long-term result is weight gain. This occurs because the body acts as if it is being starved, storing energy as fat in the cell pockets. Unfortunately, when the diet peters out, the weight piles on.

However, a happy side-effect of a detoxification programme followed by a good-quality diet is weight loss, but only in people who were overweight. Also, as the foods consumed are low in calories, any excess fat falls away – and with it all the toxins stored there!

A healing crisis

It isn't all roses, however. A detoxification diet releases toxins and debris into the bloodstream where they circulate until they reach the liver and kidneys. When the quantity of toxins exceeds the body's ability to remove them, detoxification reactions can occur, resulting in lethargy, headaches and occasionally diarrhoea.

Fortunately, the feeling of being unwell lasts for only a few days. Please don't let these possible side-effects demotivate you, however, for the ill feeling is a positive indication that the toxins are in the process of being removed. It is a sure sign that you are on your way to improved health. Drinking six to eight small glasses of pure water a day will considerably reduce the severity of the symptoms, however. I must add that many people actually suffer no adverse reactions at all.

Cleansing water

As water is required for most of what happens in our bodies, a steady intake is essential (at least eight small glasses of liquid per day). Sufficient clean water is also needed to aid detoxification – distilled water being by far the most beneficial. It not only has the ability to cleanse, it is also capable of drawing heavy metals, salts and other debris from the tissues. If you are able to obtain distilled water, it is important to note that filtered water should be used once the programme has been completed (see Chapter 8 for more information on water).

However, if you are unable to obtain distilled water for your detoxification programme, filtered water is an acceptable alternative. I would highly recommend that filtered water then be drunk for the rest of your life. If this is not possible, uncarbonated mineral water should be used. It is not the best choice, as it does not draw harmful substances from the tissues effectively, but it is superior to tap water. Note that room temperature water is more easily absorbed by the body than is chilled water.

Your 21-day detoxification programme

When you are accustomed to the new foods in your diet, you can begin the 21-day detoxification programme in earnest.

The following are important points to remember.

- Try to start your day with a glass of hot water with freshly squeezed lemon juice and maybe a little grated ginger root.
- Make fruit, vegetables, whole grains and cereals, nuts, unsaturated oils, herbs, spices and pulses the mainstay of the programme,

incorporating sea vegetables and sprouted beans, seeds and herbs if possible.

- Increase the amounts of fruit, vegetables, nuts, seeds and pulses you eat until they make up at least 50 per cent of your diet.
- Eat the above foods as regular snacks, too.
- Eat a healthy breakfast, lunch and dinner, but don't pile up the plate. If possible, consume 25 per cent of your daily intake at breakfast, 50 per cent at lunch and 25 per cent at dinnertime. (If you can't manage this, don't worry. Just make sure you don't eat too much towards the end of the day.)
- Try to cut out all dairy products apart from natural live yogurt and butter, remembering to use only a small amount of the latter.
- Eat whole grains and cereals, such as oats, barley, maize, couscous, millet, spelt, buckwheat and brown rice. Omit wheat, a common allergen, for the duration of your detoxification programme (buckwheat is not a true wheat).
- Use the recommended unsaturated oils, such as olive, hemp, corn, safflower and sunflower oils.
- Buy only organically grown produce. Most supermarkets sell it now. The superior taste makes up for the slight difference in cost.
- Drink six to eight small glasses of distilled or filtered water a day. Make up the eight to ten glasses of liquid recommended by drinking green or rooibosch tea, herbal infusions and raw fruit and vegetable juices. Be aware that fruit teas may contain flavourings.
- Have your last snack at least an hour before bedtime.
- Strive for a stress-free eating environment and never eat on your feet. Concentrate on enjoying your meals – don't watch television or read at the same time.
- Take exercise, as tolerated (see below).
- Take in some fresh air every day (see below).
- Take plenty of rest, following a deep breathing and relaxation exercise at least once a day – you may want to use a relaxation tape to help you through the process. These are available from most healthfood shops.

To achieve maximum detoxification, reduce or cut out the following.

- Dairy products and meat. If you do not wish to remove meat from the programme, remember to eat only small, lean cuts – the portions being no larger or thicker than the size of your palm. Red meat in particular takes a long time to digest, using energy that could otherwise be used by your body for detoxification. Organic tofu and other soya foods are healthy alternatives.

- White refined sugar.
- White refined flour.
- Additives, such as preservatives and colourings.
- Foods grown in a chemical environment.
- Junk food and salt.
- Fried foods.
- Microwaved foods.
- Caffeine, including coffee, caffeine teas, cola drinks, chocolate and cocoa.
- Alcohol.
- Tobacco.
- Artificial sweeteners, such as aspartame and saccharine.
- Finally, remember to take your drinks at least half an hour before and half an hour after eating. The greater the gap between eating and drinking, the less likelihood there is of important hydrochloric (stomach) acid being diluted.

Exercise and fresh air

Gentle, sustained exercise and daily fresh air are fundamental to the process of cleansing. The flow of lymph through the lymph glands – which operate as a sewage system and are heavily burdened during detoxification – is stimulated by muscular movement. It is only, therefore, by taking regular exercise that toxins are pushed to the liver and kidneys where they are neutralized prior to being eliminated from the body.

Because exercise can be very difficult for people with CFS/ME, keep it gentle. Circling your shoulders backwards and forwards several times a day will be beneficial, as will swinging your arms, turning and tilting your head, full body side-dips and side-twists and going up on tiptoe several times. Walking is good, too. You only need to walk around the house and maybe then climb the stairs two or three times more than you would normally. Remember to start any new exercise very gradually, however.

Eastern-style exercises, such as tai chi, chi kung and yoga, are specially designed to restore health, so may be worth considering at this point. Instructional video tapes can easily be purchased, enabling you to devise a personal programme suited to your own abilities and limitations.

Fresh air is equally important as toxic gases are dispelled from our bodies via the lungs. Furthermore, the inhalation of clean, fresh oxygen sustains the metabolic reactions within each cell. Don't worry if you are not able to walk too far, though, as a walk around the garden once or twice a day or a short walk along the road should provide sufficient fresh air. If walking is very difficult at this early stage, simply wrapping up warmly and standing at the open door or by an open window for a while is far better than nothing. Remember, things will get better!

Nutrition maintenance

When you have successfully completed the detoxification programme, remember to eat a wide variety of organic whole foods.

To maintain the detoxification of harmful chemicals and continue strengthening all your bodily systems, the following long-term eating habits should, ideally, be adhered to:

- continue to eat three or four small meals a day, remembering not to go hungry;
- choose organically produced foods;
- keep the high fibre content, eating fruit, vegetables, whole grains and cereals;
- have healthy food available at home or at work so you can 'snack' whenever you wish;
- eat wholemeal breads, pasta and brown rice;
- eat plenty of pulses, as well as a variety of seeds and nuts;
- keep your intake of dairy products low;
- remember to eat two to three organic soft-boiled eggs a week – vegetarians should eat four to five;
- limit consumption of red meats, especially cured and smoked meats, as a great deal of energy is used to digest them;
- eat white meat and oily fish in moderation;
- eat plenty of raw fruit and vegetables, making salads a must;
- consume at least eight glasses of liquid a day, including that in fruit and vegetable juices and green and rooibosch (redbush) tea;
- if you find it difficult to eat only the foods recommended, eat 10 per cent of your foods just for fun.

Finally, if you deviate from your diet – whether during detoxification or afterwards – try not to be disheartened. Just return to your healthy foods and forget the slight lapse. There will be times when you may prefer to put the diet aside for a while, such as when eating out or during a holiday. This doesn't mean that you've stopped your healthy diet. Take up where you left off as soon as you can and get back to improving your health.

Suggested menus

The following menus are to be used during and after the detoxification period. Note that the cup you should use for the measures given below is a small teacup or American cup measure rather than a mug. Drinks are not included.

Day 1

Breakfast:	Grapefruit and 2 slices wholemeal toast
Snack:	$\frac{1}{3}$ cup mixed sunflower seeds and almonds
Lunch:	Farmhouse Salad (see page 82)
Snack:	$\frac{1}{3}$ cup dried apricots
Dinner:	Irish Stew (see page 96)
Snack:	Two oat cakes

Day 2

Breakfast:	Porridge with cracked linseeds, raw honey and rice milk
Snack:	Banana
Lunch:	2 soft-poached eggs on wholemeal toast
Snack:	$\frac{1}{3}$ cup pecan nuts
Dinner:	Grilled chicken breast with potatoes, carrots and green beans
Snack:	Apple

Day 3

Breakfast:	Wedge of cantaloupe melon
Snack:	carob bar (available from healthfood shops)
Lunch:	Bean and Vegetable Soup (see page 87) with 2 wholemeal rolls
Snack:	$\frac{1}{3}$ cup mixed dried fruit and nuts
Dinner:	Home-made chicken curry with brown rice
Snack:	2 slices wholemeal toast

Day 4

Breakfast:	Zingy Banana (see page 76)
Snack:	2 oat cakes
Lunch:	Parsnip and Carrot Soup (see page 85)
Snack:	$\frac{1}{3}$ cup dried apricots
Dinner:	Beanburgers and No-fry Potato Chips (see pages 90 and 95)
Snack:	$\frac{1}{3}$ cup mixed nuts

Day 5

Breakfast:	Porridge with cracked linseeds, soya milk and a little muscovado sugar
Snack:	$\frac{1}{3}$ cup pecan nuts
Lunch:	Baked Mackerel with Gooseberry Sauce (see page 95)
Snack:	2 kiwi fruit
Dinner:	Mixed Vegetable Casserole (see page 89)
Snack:	2 slices wholemeal toast

Day 6

Breakfast:	Fresh Fruit Salad (see page 98)
Snack:	2 oat cakes
Lunch:	Scotch Broth (see page 84) and slice of Carob Cake (see page 100)
Snack:	$\frac{1}{3}$ cup mixed nuts
Dinner:	Falafel (similar to a veggie burger and available from healthfood shops) with salad
Snack:	Orange

Day 7

Breakfast:	2 slices wholemeal toast with raw honey
Snack:	2 rice cakes
Lunch:	Mixed salad, baked apples
Snack:	Pear
Dinner:	Baked wild salmon with potatoes, broccoli and carrots
Snack:	1 Banana and Date Muffin (see page 78)

7

Additional Health Problems Associated with CFS/ME

Unfortunately, people with CFS/ME often develop additional health problems. 'Complications' can include blood pressure that drops abnormally, a racing heartbeat, restless leg syndrome, an underactive thyroid gland, low blood sugar levels, a chronic yeast infection, food sensitivities, chemical sensitivities and adrenal exhaustion. However, the adoption of a healthy diet, the use of nutritional supplements and certain lifestyle changes can often minimize these problems. These actions may even make them disappear.

Adrenal exhaustion

Adrenal exhaustion is common in chronic illness and CFS/ME is no exception. The adrenal glands, which sit on top of the kidneys and may be thought of as the body's 'batteries', produce the adrenaline that fires the heart. However, excessive stress causes these glands to pump more adrenaline than necessary, which is obviously very draining for them.

Apart from adrenaline, the adrenal glands manufacture approximately 50 hormones and other substances that play key roles in virtually every bodily function. It makes sense then to say that adrenal exhaustion leads to problems in many areas. The stress that damages the adrenal glands in this way comes from mental, physical and emotional sources. Examples are shocks, worry, emotional upsets, lack of sleep, illness, caffeine, alcohol, smoking, drugs (both illegal and medicinal), overwork, shift work, skipped meals and rapid weight loss.

In order to treat adrenal exhaustion and low blood sugar (see below), the vicious circle of overstimulation must be broken while simultaneously repairing the damage to the adrenal glands. The chronic fatigue healing diet is of great benefit to these glands, as are the recommended supplements. However, pantothenic acid (vitamin B5) is the most useful, 500 mg daily being the therapeutic dosage. Vitamin C is also useful, at a daily dosage of 1000–3000 mg.

As well as eliminating these stressors, meditation and relaxation will make a huge difference. Siberian ginseng, which protects the body from stress, can be greatly beneficial, as can the famous Rescue Remedy – a Bach flower remedy that helps to ease shock and panic attacks. If you are experiencing a situation that is particularly stressful or have unresolved emotional issues, I strongly advise that you see a skilled counsellor.

When, finally, the adrenal glands are functioning more efficiently, virtually every system in the body will improve. Qualified nutritional consultants now offer a test that can determine if you are suffering from adrenal exhaustion.

Low blood sugar

As the adrenal glands help to control blood sugar levels, poor sugar metabolism (hypoglycaemia) is often a knock-on effect of adrenal exhaustion. When hypoglycaemia occurs, any sugar consumed will travel straight into the bloodstream, pushing up blood sugar levels, only to later make levels fall dramatically, creating a yo-yo effect. Continued bombardment of white refined sugar and caffeine will ultimately overstimulate the pancreas to produce more insulin than is required.

It is most important that a low blood sugar situation is attended to as the system may break down further – diabetes may even develop. The diet guidelines outlined in this book will aid the situation, as will pantothenic acid, the B complex vitamins and vitamin C, at the dosages given in Chapter 4.

Hypothyroidism

Poor thyroid function (hypothyroidism) is another offshoot of adrenal exhaustion and believed to be fairly common in CFS/ME. Again, I would advise that you see a nutritionist and ascertain, via a test, if adrenal exhaustion is indeed a problem. When left untreated, it can have profound consequences for health and well-being, for the thyroid gland acts as a kind of thermostat and controls the body's metabolic rate. Typical symptoms include weight gain, below normal body temperature, depression, anxiety, memory impairment, dry hair and skin, cold hands and feet and loss of libido.

Unfortunately, the standard medical laboratory test for thyroid function often indicates normal function when there is actually low output. The basal temperature test – where you take your temperature with a glass thermometer daily on waking – is a more accurate measure of thyroid activity. It should read between 36.6°C (97.8°F) and 36.8°C (98.2°F). A temperature of 36.4°C (97.4°F) or less suggests impaired function.

The prescribed medication – thyroxine – does not always improve symptoms, however. In fact, thyroxine, which is a synthetic substance, appears to be poorly used by the body. It may not be prescribed anyway without an abnormal laboratory test result.

There are numerous vitamins, minerals and amino acids that are vital to healthy thyroid function, including iodine, selenium, calcium, magnesium, vitamin A and L-Tyrosine. Thyro Complex is a special formulation containing all the above in the correct balance. Raw glandular thyroid, available as 'T-Lyph', is also recommended as a further support. Any of the adaptogenic herbs (see Chapter 4) can be considered as useful extras as they help to balance the whole endocrine system, of which both the thyroid and adrenal glands are part. The above supplements are available from healthfood shops or specialist supplement manufacturers. (See the Further Reading section for details of an excellent book about hypothyroidism.)

Candida

Yeasts live all around us. It is even normal to have a certain amount of yeast – candida albicans – inside the body, particularly within the digestive tract. Unfortunately, people with compromised immune systems, such as those with CFS/ME, are particularly susceptible to candida overgrowth, as are people who have taken repeated courses of antibiotics, steroids or use the birth control pill. The outward signs of a candida infection (candidiasis) include recurring athlete's foot, oral and/or vaginal thrush, digestive symptoms and a craving for sugar. As often there are no outward signs of candidiasis, however, it may be helpful to take a test that is offered by a qualified nutritionist.

When the immune system is too weak to combat the growing infection – as may be the case with CFS/ME – candida can spread throughout the body, in many cases even damaging the gut wall. This situation is commonly known as 'leaky gut'. Large amounts of escaped food molecules may eventually weaken the immune system, giving rise to fatigue, depression, headaches, impaired memory, digestive problems, recurrent vaginitis and cystitis, PMS, loss of libido, irritability, hypothyroidism (underactive thyroid function) and hypoglycaemia (low blood sugar). It also commonly causes food, drug and chemical sensitivities.

As many of the symptoms of candida overgrowth are the same as those of CFS/ME, it can be difficult to distinguish the two. In some sufferers, candidiasis may be the chief cause of symptoms, in which case a diet that is very low in sugar (sugar feeds candida) and yeast will help to clear the infection and alleviate symptoms. In most cases, however, specific antibiotics and/or antifungal medications are required from your doctor to tackle the condition. These should be used in conjunction with a low-sugar and low-yeast diet. (See the Further Reading section for details of a book that further describes the link between CFS/ME and candida.)

Foods to avoid	Alternatives
Cheese, including cottage and cream cheese Bread Cakes Pitta bread and buns Marmite Mushrooms Soy sauce Stock cubes Tartare sauce Bovril Vinegar Pickles Beer Wine Cider Watch out for 'leavening', 'pickled' 'fermented' and 'malt' on labels Chocolate with sugar in it (removing all forms of sugar is advised) Dried fruits Yogurt Salad dressings Ketchup Stuffing Tofu Spirits Monosodium glutamate (MSG)	Perhaps the most difficult yeast food to replace is bread. But healthfood shops now stock a sugar-, yeast-, wheat-, egg- and milk-free bread mix, to which you just add the flour of your choice. Chapatis, rye crispbreads and rice cakes. For stock, either home-made and kept frozen or vegetable bouillon paste (available in healthfood shops), broth mix, in soya cubes, all made without yeast.

Food sensitivities

Leaky gut (described above) is probably the most common cause of food sensitivity. The symptoms include fatigue, headache, dizziness, insomnia, depression or anxiety and a strong thirst, all of which arise after eating.

Discovering whether or not you are sensitive to a particular food or foods can be difficult. However, a test for leaky gut is offered by qualified nutritionists. Alternatively, a food elimination programme may be useful.

Food elimination

Although most adverse reactions to foods are a result of food 'intolerance', we often erroneously describe them as 'allergies'. The difference is that an intolerance reaction can take up to 24 hours to occur, whereas a true allergy provokes an immediate reaction. Allergic responses can vary from a headache to anaphylactic shock, which is life-threatening.

You may have a fairly good idea about which foods you are sensitive to. If not, keep a careful record of the foods you eat and note any symptoms. When you have a clearer idea of the culprits, eliminate them from your diet for a period of one month. If you want to eliminate dairy and/or wheat products, ensure that you replace the dairy products with sufficient foods that contain oil, such as oily fish, nuts, seeds and so on, and wheat products with alternative grains so that your diet does not become deficient in essential nutrients.

If you suspect you are sensitive to a large number of foods, I would advise that you attend an allergy testing clinic. There are many allergy-friendly foods and supplements available from healthfood shops, as well as certain pharmacies.

When the offending foods are first eliminated, there is occasionally a withdrawal reaction. Fatigue, headaches, twitching, and irritability are normal symptoms, and can persist for up to 15 days. Drinking as much water as possible will help to reduce these symptoms. It also aids detoxification, helping to flush any residual offending foods through the system.

A hypersensitive stage can then follow. If you then unwittingly eat a food being eliminated, the ensuing reaction can be severe, particularly when there is a true allergy.

Reintroduction strategy

Towards the end of the month, you may feel better than you have for a long time. The feeling of well-being can be so great you won't want to bother reintroducing the foods you've excluded. However, for those who do wish to reintroduce those foods, the following procedure is suggested.

- **Day 1**   In the morning, reintroduce a small amount of one of the foods eliminated (not a full-sized portion). Do the same later in the day. Record any symptoms.
- **Day 2**   If you fail to experience symptoms, repeat the exercise. Once again, record any symptoms. If you get through the second day, this is really good news!
- **Day 4**   After two days you can safely reintroduce this food into your diet on a fairly regular basis.

Repeat this four-day reintroduction procedure with each food eliminated. Any side-effects should have occurred within four days. If you do experience symptoms – say, for example, you develop a headache after reintroducing tomatoes – it would be better to leave tomatoes alone for at least six months before attempting to reintroduce them again. However, some foods may always cause an adverse reaction, so it would be wise to withdraw them from your diet altogether.

You may be disappointed, too, if your problem is a true allergy. In such instances, the offending food provokes an immediate reaction – that is, the immune system responds as if it is being invaded, setting up antibodies to the food in question. Obviously you will need to continue avoiding this food. I will just add that dairy products are the number one food allergen and wheat comes second. It might seem impossible to cut these out completely, but, as we saw earlier, you can find alternatives, such as foods containing oils in place of dairy products and other grains instead of wheat.

8

Toxic Overload

The last 50 years have seen scientific advances that could barely have been guessed at in our grandparents' day. There are vaccinations, medicines and procedures that literally save lives. There are synthetic chemicals that have caused industries to boom and made housework and personal care so much easier. It is a sad fact, however, that these marvellous advances are slowly weakening our immune systems, for we ingest a small amount of the toxins they emit every day.

Chemical sensitivities

As mentioned earlier, people with CFS/ME are particularly susceptible to chemical stressors, which enter the body through the skin, nasal passages and digestive tract. The constant onslaught of chemicals greatly stress the detoxification organs, causing sluggish liver function and impairment of the immune system. As a result, infections can linger and fatigue may persist. In time, the immune system may even begin to react against the chemicals themselves. Reactions can vary from hives, itching, skin erruptions, runny nose, sneezing, diarrhoea, tinnitus and cramps to excessive fatigue, respiratory problems and confusion.

Indoor air contaminants include building materials, paints, varnish, glues, deodorants, plastics, carpeting, insecticides, disinfectants, detergents, dyes and gas leakage from cookers and heaters. Personal care products such as deodorants, skin lotions, cosmetics, perfumes, shower gels, shampoo and conditioners and so on can also provoke adverse reactions in sensitive individuals. Biologically friendly products are now available at certain high street chemists and from some suppliers of nutritional supplements (see the Useful Addresses section for details of one such supplier).

Outdoor contaminants include industrial gases, traffic exhaust fumes, smog, crop-spraying and those created in the process of paving and resurfacing roads. Synthetic drugs – that is, those derived from petroleum – are a common source of sensitivity, too. The colourings and flavourings in medicines and foods can also cause problems.

Avoiding exposure to the chemicals that cause you the most problems will doubtless improve your condition. Following the diet recommended in this book, as well as the use of the recommended nutritional supplements, is also important and can reduce chemical sensitivity.

Organophosphates

One of the most common chemical sensitivities is to organophosphates (known as OPs), which are now widely used in farming practices throughout the Western world. OPs are highly toxic chemicals used for pest control in crop production and animal husbandry as a matter of course. They are also used in home pesticides, such as fly sprays. Originally developed to attack the central nervous system in order to kill for the purposes of warfare, they can adversely affect every system in the body and are believed to be implicated in the onset of CFS/ME. OPs are never used in organic farming, however.

Typical symptoms of OP poisoning include mental and physical fatigue, poor muscle stamina, muscle pain, drug intolerance, irritable bowel syndrome, sweating, low body temperature, numb patches, muscle twitching, clumsiness, mood swings, irritability, poor short-term memory and poor concentration. Many people with CFS/ME display all these symptoms.

The detoxification of OPs can be promoted by avoiding exposure to them, by following an organic diet and taking antioxidant supplements. Vitamins A, C and E, B12, magnesium and selenium are particularly effective.

Heavy metals

Besides chemicals, our bodies are absorbing small quantities of heavy metals every day. Hair mineral analysis, which can be organized by a qualified nutritionist, can show high levels of minerals in the body. The worst culprits are the following.

Aluminium

As high levels of aluminium in the body cause damage to the central nervous system, it is believed to be highly implicated in the evolution and persistence of CFS/ME.

Sources of aluminium poisoning may be aluminium cookware,

foil, containers and underarm deodorants. This metal can also be found in coffee, bleached white flour and some antacid medicines.

Interestingly, experts now believe that magnesium and calcium deficiencies increase the toxic effects of ingested aluminium.

Mercury

Those with amalgam tooth fillings are ingesting minute amounts of mercury vapour every day and mercury is the second most toxic heavy metal in the world. The leaked mercury vapour can gradually weaken the immune system, causing many of the symptoms of CFS/ME.

Synthetic white fillings are a safe alternative.

Lead

Ingested lead is known to cause neurological and psychological disturbances. Some old houses still have lead piping, others have copper piping that was joined together with lead-based solder.

The use of a water filter is highly recommended in cases like this, although, obviously, replacing the old piping with modern copper or synthetic piping makes things far safer.

Cadmium

High carbohydrate consumption is now thought to be linked with high cadmium levels in the body. Smoking cigarettes is another cause of cadmium buildup – cadmium being mainly absorbed by the lungs. This metal is known to be damaging to the kidneys and lungs. It can, however, be gradually removed by a detoxification diet, followed by good nutrition.

Water

Experts believe that the thirst reflex may be suppressed in people with CFS/ME, leading to the intake of fluids being insufficient to supply all the body needs. In addition, live blood microscopy has shown that the red blood cells of those with CFS/ME become sticky and clump together, which emphasizes the need for adequate water consumption. However, whether or not tap water is suitable for human consumption is a matter for debate. Water in the UK is thought to be superior to that of a number of other countries. It is still laden with toxic chemicals and inorganic salts that are undoubtedly detrimental to people with CFS/ME, however.

In areas of hard water, where rainwater has run through limestone (containing sodium salts and calcium salts), our tap water has a high mineral content, particularly of mineral salts. This can cause fluid retention and a concentration of salts in our tissues. Ultimately, it can even lead to high blood pressure and hardening of the arteries. Soft water, on the other hand, is usually filtered through sandstone and peat, which removes many of the impurities. This is better, until chemicals are added, such as chlorine and, in some areas, fluoride.

Our water is taken from the following sources:

- **Reservoirs** The chemicals mentioned above are added to this surface water.
- **Deep artesian wells** Water from these wells is the purest of all and is added to reservoir water.
- **Ground water** The high levels of suspended matter and dissolved acids give ground water its brown colour, so aluminium sulphate is added as a coagulant, then chemical polyelectrolytes are put in to further settle the coagulated waste and, although this water is then passed through sand filters to remove the settled particles, many of the chemicals remain; this water is then added to reservoir water.

As you can see, our tap water can end up being saturated with inappropriate mineral salts and added chemicals. Other pollutants that often seep in then contaminate it further. If you are interested in what the water is like in your postal area, the water authority will provide a breakdown on request. However, as tap water is certainly of some detriment to people with CFS/ME, I recommend the use of purified water.

Types of purified water recommended are the following.

- **Distilled water** Water is distilled by boiling and condensing the steam. This very pure water successfully leeches excessive minerals and other salts from the body, but it must only be used for periods of up to six months, otherwise necessary minerals risk being removed. For maximum effect, drink water every hour, but not more than one glass. Try to drink a total of eight small glasses a day. The results can be spectacular when used in conjunction with the detoxification diet (see Chapter 6). However, retailers of distilled water are thin on the ground (see the Useful Addresses section for details of suppliers of water distillers).
- **Filtered water** Although distilled water has superior effects

during the detoxification diet, filtered water should be used to stay healthy afterwards. Water filters on the market vary from simple carbon filters to carbon filters with silver mesh components that even destroy bacteria. There are also reverse osmosis filters, which produce very clean water while still retaining some of the precious trace minerals. It must be said, however, that their individual effectiveness at removing pollutants is proportionate to their cost. Don't let this put you off, though, as an inexpensive carbon filter is far better than no filter at all.

- **Spring water** Bottled spring water may be used, if desired. However, use types that are uncarbonated and low in sodium.

Note that purified water should be used to make drinks and wash fruit and vegetables.

Microwave ovens

Although microwave ovens can save much time and energy for people with CFS/ME, there is evidence that their use can depress the immune system. Microwaves heat food by vibrating the molecules of the food together to produce heat. However, this process damages food at the DNA level, which, in turn, damages bodily DNA. I strongly advise, therefore, that you use a microwave oven only when you feel too unwell to use more conventional methods of cooking.

As you can see, there are many toxic substances that, over time, depress the immune system and are undoubtedly a problem for people with CFS/ME. When you remove as many of these substances as possible from your diet and local environment, there are bound to be improvements.

PART TWO

Healing Recipes

The ingredients used in the following recipes should be organic, if possible. Any water used should be filtered.

ESSENTIAL BASICS

Home-made Vegetable Stock

1 tsp sunflower oil	4 parsley stalks
1 potato, chopped	1 sprig thyme
1 carrot, chopped	1 bay leaf
1 celery stick, chopped	pinch freshly ground black
1 onion, chopped	pepper
2 garlic cloves	900 ml (1½ pints) filtered water

Heat the sunflower oil in a large saucepan, then add the vegetables. Cover and sauté very gently for about 10 minutes. Add the herbs, mix and then pour the water into the pan. Bring back to the boil, then simmer very gently, partially covered, for 40 minutes, until a concentrate forms (you will have about 600 ml/1 pint of liquid left). Strain, season with the pepper and use as required. This stock will add flavour to stews and soups or may simply be poured over steamed vegetables. It can be frozen or stored in a refrigerator for three to four days.

Shortcrust Potato Pastry

Makes 225 g ($\frac{1}{2}$ lb) pastry

75 g (3 oz) rice flour
50 g (2 oz) cornflour
small pinch sea salt
175 g (6 oz) cooked potatoes,
  mashed

100 g (4 oz) organic unsalted
  butter, cut into thin slices

Beat the flours and salt into the potato. Add the butter and beat into the mixture. Work into a ball, wrap in clingfilm and refrigerate for 30 minutes. Knead the dough on a floured surface, forming the required shape. Due to its high butter content, this pastry should be used sparingly.

Shortcrust Pastry

Makes 225 g ($\frac{1}{2}$ lb) pastry

1 large banana
1 egg yolk
2 tbsp filtered water
75 g (3 oz) rice flour
75 g (3 oz) cornflour

65 g ($2\frac{1}{2}$ oz) organic unsalted
  butter
65 g ($2\frac{1}{2}$ fl oz) olive oil
small pinch sea salt

Beat the banana to a smooth purée with the egg yolk and water. Sift the flours into a bowl, adding the butter and olive oil. Rub to form fine crumbs. Mix in the purée and salt, using a knife. Work the dough into a ball, wrap in clingfilm and refrigerate for 30 minutes. Knead on a floured surface, then refrigerate for another 30 minutes before rolling out to the required shape.

BREAKFASTS

Muesli

Serves 1

1 tbsp organic rolled oats
$\frac{1}{2}$ dspn oat germ
85 ml (3 fl oz) soya milk or
   rice milk
1 dspn organic natural live
   yogurt

$\frac{1}{2}$ tbsp raw honey
$\frac{1}{2}$ tbsp lemon juice
$\frac{1}{4}$ tbsp linseeds, ground
$\frac{1}{4}$ tbsp almond, ground
1 apple, grated

Soak the rolled oats and oat germ in the milk overnight. Stir in the yogurt, honey and lemon juice the next morning. Sprinkle with the ground linseeds and almonds and top with the grated apple. Serve.

Zingy Banana

Serves 1

2–3 bananas, mashed
juice of 1 lemon
pinch ground cinnamon
chopped nuts, any type (optional)

Add the lemon juice to the mashed banana. If necessary, add a little filtered water to make a smooth, thick sauce. Garnish with the cinnamon. Sprinkle on the chopped nuts. Serve.

Warming Porridge

Serves 6

1.2 l (2 pints) filtered water
150 g (5 oz) medium porridge
  oats
200 ml (7 fl oz) soya milk,
  plus more if required

1 tbsp raw honey or as
  required
1 tbsp cracked linseeds

Pour the water into a large saucepan and bring to the boil. As it reaches boiling point, sprinkle in the porridge oats in a steady rain, stirring all the time with a wooden spoon or a fork. When the porridge thickens, lower the heat, cover and simmer, very gently, for 10 to 15 minutes, stirring from time to time, adding more water if it becomes too stiff. Pour into warm bowls and add the required amount of soya milk and honey. Mix in the cracked linseeds and serve.

Cinnamon Compote

Serves 4

25 g (1 oz) dried apricots
25 g (1 oz) dried apples
25 g (1 oz) dried peaches
40 g (1½ oz) dried figs
1 cinnamon stick

300 ml (½ pint) orange juice
25 g (1 oz) pears
2 tbsp organic live yogurt
4 tsp sesame seeds, toasted

Soak the dried fruit and cinnamon stick in the orange juice overnight. The next day, peel and chop the pears and put the pieces into a saucepan together with the soaked fruit, juice and cinnamon stick, heat gently and simmer gently for 15 minutes. Serve hot, topped with the yogurt and toasted sesame seeds.

Banana and Date Muffins

Serves 2

2 wholemeal muffins
2 bananas
1 tbsp chopped dates
2 tsp sesame seeds

Slice the muffins in half and toast them. Mash the bananas with a fork and stir in the chopped dates and sesame seeds. Spread this mixture over the muffins and serve.

Poached Eggs on Granary Bread

Serves 2

4 slices Granary bread, toasted
2 eggs
4 tomatoes, halved

25 g (1 oz) unsalted organic butter

Cut the toast into triangles. Soft-poach the eggs and grill the tomatoes. Spread the butter sparingly on the toast and top with the eggs and tomatoes. Serve.

SALADS

Tangy Mayonnaise

Makes 350 g (12 oz)

350 g (12 oz) tofu
4 tbsp soya milk
4 tbsp freshly squeezed lemon
* juice*

2 tbsp olive oil
½ tsp sea salt

Place all the ingredients in a blender and mix well. Serve. May be used as a dressing with potatoes, fish, grains, salads, vegetables and so on.

Raw Beetroot Salad

Serves 2

1 raw beetroot, finely grated
1 tsp raw honey
1 tsp lemon juice

Place all the ingredients in a bowl and mix well. Refrigerate for 1 hour, then eat like a coleslaw with a salad or other food. This salad will keep in a jar in the fridge for a few days.

Eggless Egg Salad

Serves 4

750 g (1½ lbs) tofu, pressed for
   half an hour, then mashed
   with a fork
1 celery stick, finely chopped
1 small onion or 3–4 spring
   onions, chopped

1 tbsp natural soy sauce
8 tbsp Tangy Mayonnaise (see
   recipe, above)
1 tsp ground turmeric

Mix all the ingredients together with a fork. Serve with a baked potato or salad.

Apple and Avocado Salad

Serves 6

2 large red dessert apples,
   cored, quartered and diced
1 ripe avocado, peeled and
   diced
2 celery sticks, chopped
50 g (2 oz) sultanas
50 g (2 oz) walnuts, chopped
150 g (6 oz) sweetcorn

75 g (3 oz) Cheshire cheese,
   crumbled
100 g (4 oz) organic natural
   live yogurt
2 tbsp apple juice
1 tbsp fresh mint, chopped
1 lettuce

Place the apples, avocado, celery, sultanas, walnuts, sweetcorn and cheese together in a bowl and mix. Blend the remaining ingredients, except the lettuce, together in a separate bowl, then pour over the salad and mix to combine. Line six small dishes with lettuce leaves and fill with the salad. Serve.

Lunchtime Salad

Serves 2

1 pear, peeled, cored and
  chopped
2 tbsp fresh lemon juice
2 carrots, grated
175 g (6 oz) cucumber,
  chopped
100 g (4 oz) white cabbage,
  shredded

100 g (4 oz) low-fat cheese,
  diced
75 g (3 oz) organic natural
  live yogurt
2 tbsp low-fat mayonnaise
pinch dried mixed herbs
2 tomatoes, cut into wedges

Coat the chopped pear with the lemon juice, then mix with the vegetables and cheese. Mix together the yogurt, mayonnaise and herbs. Pour over the salad and arrange the tomato wedges around the edge. Serve with wholemeal bread rolls.

Farmhouse Salad

Serves 4

1 Cos lettuce, washed and
  shaken
1 iceberg lettuce, washed and
  shaken
1 bunch spring onions, white
  parts cut finely lengthways,
  green parts discarded

1 cucumber, peeled and
  chopped
6 radishes, thinly sliced

DRESSING

1 tbsp lemon juice
pinch demerara sugar
small pinch sea salt
1 tsp English mustard
4 tbsp olive oil

Place the lettuce in a large salad bowl. Add the cucumber, radishes and onions. Place all the dressing ingredients except the oil in a bowl. Stir together, gradually beating in the oil to give a smooth texture. Mix into the salad. Serve.

SOUPS

Lentil, Vegetable and Millet Soup

Serves 6

Submitted by Susan Thorpe

2 medium onions, chopped
pinch sea salt or to taste
2 tbsp olive oil
3–4 garlic cloves or to taste, crushed
2–3 carrots, chopped
2 celery sticks, chopped
pinch dried mixed herbs
2 tsp garam masala (optional)
1 tbsp stoneground organic wholemeal flour
1 tbsp tomato purée
2–3 tomatoes, skinned and roughly chopped (immerse in boiling water for a minute or two to aid skinning)

100 g (4 oz) organic lentils (green, brown or mixed) soaked in water for a minimum of 30 minutes, then strained
1.2 l (2 pints) vegetable stock or Home-made Vegetable Stock with 600 ml (1 pint) water added (see page 74)
40 g (1$\frac{1}{2}$–2 oz) millet or pasta
150 g (5 oz) cabbage, chopped
150 g (5 oz) broccoli or cauliflower, cut into small florets
100 g (4 oz) mushrooms, chopped
splash shoyu (organic soy sauce) (optional)

Place the onions in a large saucepan, add salt and sauté in the olive oil for about 5 minutes. Add the garlic, carrots and celery and continue cooking gently for another 5 minutes. Add the herbs and garam masala, if using, and mix well. Add the flour, mix well and cook for another minute, stirring continuously. Add the tomato purée, tomatoes, lentils and stock, mix well and simmer gently for 10 minutes. Add the millet or pasta, cabbage, broccoli or cauliflower and mushrooms and the shoyu, if using, then stir thoroughly. Bring to the boil and simmer gently for a further 20 minutes. Serve.

Scotch Broth

Serves 4–6

750 g (1½ lbs) lean shin beef, diced
2.25 l (4 pints) filtered water
1 carrot, chopped
1 medium turnip, chopped

1 onion, chopped
2 leeks, chopped
3 tbsp pearl barley
4 sprigs fresh parsley, chopped

Place the meat and water in a large saucepan. Bring to the boil, cover and simmer for 30 minutes. Add the vegetables and barley. Simmer for another hour until all the ingredients are soft. Skim off any fat and garnish with the parsley before serving.

Spicy Lentil Soup

Serves 2

15 g (½ oz) organic unsalted butter
1 onion, chopped
1 garlic clove, crushed
2 tsp ground cumin
1 tsp ground ginger
1 red pepper, deseeded and chopped
1 green pepper, deseeded and chopped

1 bay leaf
175 g (6 oz) split red lentils
600 ml (1 pint) Home-made Vegetable Stock (see page 74) or vegetable bouillon
450 ml (¾ pint) soya milk
2 sprigs fresh coriander leaves, to garnish

Melt the butter in a medium saucepan, add the onion and sauté until soft. Add the garlic and spices and sauté for a further minute, stirring all the time. Stir in the peppers, bay leaf, lentils and stock. Bring to the boil, cover and simmer for 15 minutes or until the lentils have become soft. Remove and discard the bay leaf. Stir in the soya milk and reheat without boiling. Garnish with the coriander and serve with wholemeal rolls.

Parsnip and Carrot Soup

Serves 4

350 g (12 oz) carrots, diced
350 g (12 oz) parsnips, diced
1 onion, chopped
600 ml (1 pint) Home-made
  Vegetable Stock (see page
  74)

3 tbsp peanut butter
600 ml (1 pint) soya milk
4 tsp organic natural live
  yogurt
4 sprigs fresh parsley, to
  garnish

Place the vegetables in a large saucepan with the stock and peanut butter. Bring to the boil, cover and simmer for 15 minutes. Liquidize half of the soup, then stir this into the remainder with the soya milk and reheat. Serve topped with a swirl of the yogurt and a sprig of parsley.

Parsley Soup

Serves 4

100 g (4 oz) fresh parsley,
  washed and chopped
1 onion, chopped
1 potato, diced
1 garlic clove, crushed
450 ml ($\frac{3}{4}$ pint) Home-made
  Vegetable Stock (see page
  74)

25 g (1 oz) cornflour
300 ml ($\frac{1}{2}$ pint) soya milk
pinch sea salt or to taste
pinch freshly ground black
  pepper or to taste

Place the parsley, onion, potato and garlic in a medium saucepan together with the stock and bring to the boil. Cover and simmer gently for 20 minutes. Remove from the heat and allow to cool. Liquidize until smooth, then return to the heat. Blend the cornflour with a little of the soya milk, add the remaining milk, then pour into the soup, stirring continuously until it has thickened. Season to taste with salt and pepper. Serve hot or chilled.

Golden Broth

Serves 6

1.2 l (2 pints) chicken stock or
  Home-made Vegetable Stock
  with 600 ml (1 pint) water
  added (see page 74)
1 onion, chopped
1 garlic clove
2 sprigs fresh parsley
2 sprigs fresh thyme

2 sprigs fresh mint
2 sprigs fresh lemon balm
12 coriander seeds
large pinch saffron
4 cloves
pinch sea salt or to taste
pinch freshly ground black
  pepper or to taste

Place all the ingredients in a large saucepan and bring to the boil. Simmer very gently for 30 minutes, covered, to infuse the broth with all the delicate herbal and spicy flavours. Strain and serve hot, with freshly made fingers of wholemeal toast to dip into the broth.

Leek and Fennel Soup

Serves 4–5

2 tbsp olive oil
3 leeks, washed and sliced
2 fennel bulbs, chopped
2 garlic cloves, crushed
1 tsp fennel seeds
750 ml (1¼ pints) vegetable
  stock or Home-made
  Vegetable Stock with 150 ml
  (¼ pint) water added (see
  page 74)

2 tbsp lemon juice
pinch sea salt or to taste
pinch freshly ground black
  pepper or to taste

Heat the olive oil in a large saucepan and gently sauté the leeks, fennel, garlic and fennel seeds for about 5 minutes. Add the stock and bring to the boil. Reduce the heat, cover and simmer for about 20 minutes. Purée the soup in batches. Add the lemon juice and salt and pepper, then serve.

Courgette and Cumin Soup

Serves 4

25 g (1 oz) organic unsalted
  butter
1 onion, chopped
1 garlic clove, crushed
150 g (5 oz) potatoes, peeled
  and diced
350 g ($\frac{3}{4}$ lb) courgettes, thinly
  sliced

450 ml ($\frac{3}{4}$ pint) chicken stock
  or Home-made Vegetable
  Stock (see page 74)
300 ml ($\frac{1}{2}$ pint) soya milk
1 tsp ground cumin
pinch freshly ground black
  pepper

Melt the butter in a large saucepan and add the onion and garlic. Sauté for 5 minutes, until soft. Add the cumin, then stir in the potatoes and most of the courgettes. Cook gently for 2 minutes. Add the stock, milk and pepper and bring to the boil. Cover and simmer for a further 15 minutes, until the vegetables have softened. Purée the soup. Serve, garnished with the remaining thin slices of courgette.

Bean and Vegetable Soup

Serves 4–6

25 g (1 oz) organic unsalted
  butter
225 g (8 oz) carrots, diced
225 g (8 oz) parsnips, diced
1 onion, sliced
2 potatoes, peeled and diced
1 green pepper, deseeded and
  diced
50 g (2 oz) lentils

450 ml ($\frac{3}{4}$ pint) vegetable stock
  or Home-made Vegetable
  Stock (see page 74)
450 ml ($\frac{3}{4}$ pint) soya milk
1 bouquet garni
220-g ($7\frac{1}{2}$-oz) tin red kidney
  beans, drained
220-g ($7\frac{1}{2}$-oz) tin butter beans,
  drained
4–6 sprigs fresh parsley

Melt the butter in a large frying pan and add the vegetables. Sauté for 5 minutes or until they have softened. Add the lentils, stock, soya milk and bouquet garni, bring to the boil, cover and simmer for 15–20 minutes. Remove and discard the bouquet garni. Add the beans and heat through. Serve garnished with the sprigs of parsley.

MAIN MEALS

Creamy Mushroom and Tomato Pasta

Serves 3–4

*1 tbsp olive oil, plus more if
  required*
2 garlic cloves, crushed
1 onion, diced
*375 g (13 oz) mushrooms,
  diced*
*1 large red pepper, deseeded
  and diced*

15 g ($\frac{1}{2}$ oz) cornflour
120 ml (4 fl oz) soya milk
1 tomato, diced
2 tbsp tomato purée
100 g (4 oz) fresh parsley
*450 g (1 lb) spiral pasta,
  cooked according to
  instructions on packaging*

Place the oil in a large frying pan and warm. Add the garlic, onion, mushrooms and red pepper and sauté for 5 minutes. Stir the cornflour into the soya milk. Add to the pan and stir until the mixture thickens slightly. Add the tomato, the tomato purée and parsley and stir well. Finally, add the cooked pasta and stir until heated through, adding either a little water or more flour until the desired consistency is reached. Serve.

Mixed Vegetable Casserole

Serves 4

1 aubergine, cut into 2.5-cm
(1-in) pieces
4 courgettes, cut into 1-cm
($\frac{1}{2}$-in) pieces
2 onions, finely chopped
450 g (1 lb) potatoes, cut into
2.5-cm (1-in) pieces
100 g (4 oz) okra, cut in half
lengthways
225 g (8 oz) frozen or fresh
peas
225 g (8 oz) green beans, cut
into 2.5-cm (1-in) pieces

1 red pepper, deseeded and
sliced
400-g (14-oz) tin chopped
tomatoes
300 ml ($\frac{1}{2}$ pint) vegetable stock
or Home-made Vegetable
Stock (see page 74)
4 tbsp olive oil
8 sprigs fresh parsley, chopped
1 tsp paprika

FOR THE TOPPING

3 tomatoes, sliced
1 courgette, sliced

Preheat the oven to 190°C/375°F. Place all the prepared vegetables in a large casserole dish. Add the tinned tomatoes, stock, olive oil and parsley. Mix well, then level the mixture. Arrange the tomato and courgette slices on top, alternating the slices for a decorative effect. Cover and cook in the preheated oven for 40–50 minutes, until the vegetables have softened. Serve.

No-fry Potato Chips

Serves 3

2 potatoes, peeled and chipped
1 tbsp olive oil, plus extra for greasing
$\frac{1}{2}$ tsp garlic salt

Preheat the oven to 190°C/375°F. Grease a baking sheet with a little oil. Place the chips on the prepared baking sheet and brush them with the olive oil. Sprinkle half the garlic salt over them and bake them in the preheated oven for 20 minutes. Turn the chips over, sprinkle the remaining garlic salt over them and bake for another 10 minutes. Serve hot.

Cajun Fish Fillets

Serves 4

450 g (1 lb) any white fish fillets
1 tsp cajun spice
1 tbsp paprika
pinch freshly ground black pepper or to taste
1 lemon, quartered, to garnish

Arrange the fillets on a lightly oiled grill tray. Mix together the cajun spice and paprika and sprinkle heavily over the fillets. Grill them close to the flame for 5–6 minutes or until the spices have browned and the fish is firm and will flake with a fork. Season with the black pepper and serve with a salad or the No-fry Potato Chips (see above). Garnish with the lemon wedges.

Tahini Couscous with Vegetables

Serves 4

200 ml (7 fl oz) filtered water
2½ tbsp tahini
2 garlic cloves, crushed
1 baby courgette, halved
  lengthways then sliced
2 celery sticks, thinly sliced

4–5 large crimini mushrooms,
  chopped
½ green onion, finely chopped
100 g (4 oz) couscous
1 tbsp lemon juice

Place the water, tahini, garlic, courgette and celery in a medium saucepan and bring to the boil. Simmer for 3–4 minutes. Add the mushrooms and green onion and simmer for 2 more minutes. Add the couscous and lemon juice, then stir constantly for 1 minute. Remove from the heat and cover. Allow to stand for 10–15 minutes, fluff with a fork and mix well. Serve.

Stuffed Marrow

Serves 2–3

25 g (1 oz) organic unsalted
  butter
100 g (4 oz) turnip, peeled
  and chopped
175 g (6 oz) aubergine, cubed
2 parsnips, peeled and
  chopped
2 carrots, chopped
100 g (4 oz) swede, peeled and
  chopped

1 tbsp fresh parsley, chopped
1 tsp tomato purée
450 ml (¾ pint) vegetable
  bouillon or Home-made
  Vegetable Stock (see page
  74)
550 g (1¼ lbs) marrow, peeled,
  halved lengthways and
  deseeded

Preheat the oven to 190°C/375°F. Place the butter in a large frying pan, add the prepared vegetables, except the marrow, and sauté for 5 minutes. Add the parsley, tomato purée and stock. Gently simmer for 10 minutes. Fill one half of the marrow with the mixture. Top with the other half of the marrow and wrap in foil. Bake in the preheated oven for about 35–45 minutes. Serve cut into slices.

Peppers with Tarragon

Serves 2–3

1 red pepper, deseeded and
  quartered
1 green pepper, deseeded and
  quartered
1 large garlic clove, chopped
juice of 1 lemon

2 tbsp fresh tarragon, finely
  chopped
pinch sea salt or to taste
pinch freshly ground black
  pepper or to taste
3 tbsp olive oil

Place the peppers on a grill pan and grill for 3–5 minutes, skin-side up. Leave to cool. Now remove the skin and cut the flesh of the peppers into strips. Mix together the garlic, lemon juice, most of the tarragon, salt and pepper and sprinkle over the peppers. Trickle the olive oil over and garnish with the remaining tarragon.

Tofu Spinach Quiche

Makes 1 quiche

PASTRY
> *450 g (1 lb) stoneground organic wholemeal flour*
> *4–5 tbsp olive oil*
> *pinch sea salt or to taste*
> *1 tbsp cold filtered water or as required*

FILLING
> *2 onions, diced*
> *150 ml ($\frac{1}{4}$ pint) olive oil*
> *2 tbsp fresh dill*
> *2 tbsp fresh parsley, chopped*
> *175 g (6 oz) spinach, precooked and chopped*
> *pinch sea salt*
> *450 g (1 lb) tofu*
> *4 tbsp soya milk, if necessary*

Preheat the oven to 190°C/375°F. Lightly grease a 20-cm (8-in) flan dish. Combine the pastry ingredients and knead the dough, adding water if required. Roll out the pastry on a floured surface and press into the prepared flan dish. To make the filling, place the onions and olive oil in a medium saucepan and sauté until transparent. Add the dill, parsley, cooked spinach and salt and mix well. Blend the tofu in a liquidizer, adding soya milk if it is difficult to blend on its own. Pour over the vegetable mixture and mix thoroughly. Place in the pastry case and bake in the preheated oven for about 30 minutes.

Pasta with Chicken and Beans

Serves 2

100 g (4 oz) dried penne pasta
  (or other tube pasta)
400-g (14-oz) tin tomatoes,
  roughly chopped
220-g (7½-oz) tin cut green
  beans, drained

220-g (7½-oz) tin flageolet
  beans, drained
150 g (5 oz) cooked chicken,
  cubed
50 g (2 oz) low-fat Mozzarella
  cheese, shredded

Cook the pasta according to the directions on the packaging, then drain. Combine the undrained tomatoes, green beans and flageolet beans in a large frying pan. Bring to the boil. Stir in the chicken and pasta. Heat through. Transfer to a serving dish and sprinkle with the cheese.

Hot Spinach and Vegetables with Rice

Serves 4

Submitted by David Craggs-Hinton

1.75 l (3 pints) water
450 g (1 lb) brown rice
450 g (1 lb) fresh spinach,
  chopped
25 g (1 oz) carrots, chopped
25 g (1 oz) potatoes, chopped
25 g (1 oz) aubergine, chopped
25 g (1 oz) cabbage, chopped
25 g (1 oz) French beans

50 g (2 oz) tomatoes
1 onion, sliced
3 green chillies, very finely
  chopped
pinch ground ginger
pinch ground turmeric
1 tsp ground coriander
pinch sea salt or to taste
150 ml (5 fl oz) filtered water

Bring the water to the boil in a large saucepan, pour in the rice, bring back to the boil, then reduce the heat, cover and simmer for 25–30 minutes. While the rice is cooking, mix all the remaining ingredients together in another large saucepan and bring to the boil. Simmer until the vegetables have softened (about 20 minutes). Remove from the heat and mash coarsely. Reheat and cook for 3–4 minutes, until the mixture has thickened slightly. Serve on a ring of the rice.

Beanburgers

Makes 8 burgers

440-g (15½-oz) tin red kidney
beans, drained and rinsed
1 large red onion, finely
chopped
2 sprigs fresh basil, finely
chopped

2 tsp sweet chilli sauce
1 egg, beaten
25 g (1 oz) plain organic
wholemeal flour, plus extra
to dust
2 tsp olive oil

Place the beans in a bowl and mash lightly. Add the onion, basil, chilli sauce and the egg. Mix until all the ingredients are combined. Add the flour, keeping back a little. Pat the mixture into 8 burger shapes and dust with the remaining flour. Lightly coat with the olive oil and grill under a medium heat for about 5 minutes each side. Serve with a salad, baked potato or No-fry Potato Chips (see page 90).

Baked Mackerel with Gooseberry Sauce

Serves 4

15 g (½ oz) organic unsalted butter
225 g (8 oz) gooseberries, topped and tailed
4 x 350-g (12-oz) mackerel, cleaned and heads removed
4 tsp lemon juice
1 egg, beaten

Melt the butter in a medium-sized saucepan and add the gooseberries. Cover tightly and cook over a low heat, shaking the pan occasionally, until the fruit is tender. Meanwhile, sprinkle the cavity of each fish with 1 teaspoonful of the lemon juice. Make two or three slashes in the skin on each side of the fish, then grill for 15–20 minutes, depending on the size, turning once, until tender. Purée the gooseberries and sieve to remove the pips. Pour the purée into a clean pan, beat in the egg, then reheat gently, stirring well. Place the mackerel on warmed serving plates and spoon the sauce beside them.

Irish Stew

Serves 4

750 g (1½ lbs) lamb cutlets,
  trimmed
2 onions, sliced
450 g (1 lb) potatoes, thinly
  sliced

1 tbsp fresh parsley, chopped,
  plus extra to garnish
1 tbsp fresh thyme, chopped
300 ml (½ pint) filtered water

Preheat the oven to 170°C/325°F. Layer the meat, vegetables and herbs in a deep casserole dish that has a lid, ending with a top layer of potato slices. Pour the water over and cover the dish with greaseproof paper. Cover with the lid and bake in the preheated oven for 2 hours or until tender. Serve hot, garnished with the remaining chopped parsley.

Chicken Vegetable Medley

Serves 1

juice of 2 lemons
pinch sea salt or to taste
pinch freshly ground black
  pepper or to taste
2 tsp olive oil
100-g (4-oz) skinless, boneless
  chicken breast

1 small courgette cut into
  strips
50 g (2 oz) red pepper, cut
  into strips
1 tbsp fresh parsley, chopped

Place the lemon juice, salt, pepper and half of the olive oil in a bowl, add the chicken breast and marinate for 30 minutes. Drain and grill the chicken breast until lightly browned (about 10–15 minutes). Place the remaining olive oil in a frying pan and sauté the vegetables for 15 minutes or until soft. Sprinkle the parsley over the vegetables. Cut the chicken into two pieces and place on a warmed plate. Add the vegetables. Serve.

DESSERTS

Figgy Apples

Serves 4

4 large cooking apples, peeled
   and cored
75 g (3 oz) dried figs, chopped
1 tbsp lemon juice

1 tbsp raw honey
4 tbsp apple juice
8 tbsp organic natural live
   yogurt

Preheat the oven to 180°C/350°F. Make a shallow cut around the middle of each apple, then place in a lightly oiled ovenproof dish. Place the figs, lemon juice and honey in a small pan and heat gently, stirring until well blended. Use this mixture to fill the apple cavities, pressing it down firmly, then pour the apple juice over them. Bake in the preheated oven for 45–55 minutes, until soft. Serve hot, spooning 2 tablespoons of yogurt on to each serving.

Summer Fruit Fool

Serves 4–6

175 g (6 oz) strawberries,
   hulled
175 g (6 oz) raspberries
175 g (6 oz) blueberries

125 g (4 oz) organic natural
   live yogurt
2 tsp raw honey
4–6 sprigs fresh mint, to
   garnish

Place all the ingredients, except the mint, in a blender and mix until smooth. Spoon into bowls and refrigerate until ready to serve. Garnish each serving with a sprig of mint.

Dried Fruit Compote

Serves 4

350 ml (12 oz) mixed dried
  fruits, such as apples, pears,
  prunes, peaches, apricots
1 cinnamon stick
300 ml ($\frac{1}{2}$ pint) filtered water

65 g ($2\frac{1}{2}$ oz) raisins, washed
2 tsp raw honey
juice of 1 lemon
6–8 fresh mint leaves, to
  garnish

Place the dried fruit in a large saucepan with the cinnamon and water. Heat to almost boiling, then cover and simmer gently for 12–15 minutes, until the fruit has softened. Remove from heat, add the raisins and honey and stir. Cover and leave to cool. When cool, remove the cinnamon stick and stir in the lemon juice. Transfer the compote to a serving bowl, cover with clingfilm and place in the refrigerator until required. Before serving, allow the compote to return to room temperature. Garnish with the mint leaves.

Fresh Fruit Salad

Serves 6

16–20 strawberries, hulled and
  halved
2 apples, peeled, cored and
  chopped
2 oranges, peeled and
  segmented

2 peaches, peeled and thickly
  sliced
2 tbsp fresh lemon juice
6–8 fresh mint leaves, to
  garnish (optional)

Place all the fruit in a small bowl, adding juice created during preparation, too. Mix in the lemon juice. Serve, garnished with the mint leaves, if using.

Easy Christmas Pudding

Serves 6

50 g (2 oz) apple, grated
65 g (2½ oz) apricots, chopped
65 g (2½ oz) dried dates, chopped
4 medium free-range organic eggs, beaten
120 g (4½ oz) demerara sugar
75 g (3 oz) carob flour (sometimes called carob powder)

large pinch ground mixed spice
large pinch ground cinnamon
finely grated zest of ½ a lemon
finely grated zest of ½ an orange
filtered water as required

Place all the ingredients in a large bowl and mix well. Add a little filtered water if necessary until the right consistency is reached – not too runny. Pour the mixture into 6 individual well-oiled pudding basins. Place a disk of greaseproof paper on top of the mixture of each pudding, then cover the tops securely with foil. Steam for 2 hours, checking the water regularly to ensure that the pan doesn't boil dry. Serve.

BAKING

Carob Cake

Makes one 20-cm (8-in) cake

Submitted by Susan Thorpe

*3 medium organic free-range
  eggs*
3 tbsp raw honey
*150 g (5 oz) organic
  stoneground wholemeal flour*

*25 g (1 oz) carob flour
  (sometimes called carob
  powder)*
100 g (4 oz) dried dates
2 tsp desiccated coconut

Preheat the oven to 180°C/350°F and grease and line a 20-cm (8-in) cake tin. Place the eggs and honey in a blender and combine. Mix the two types of flour together, then add gradually to the egg and honey mixture, whisking well between additions. When thoroughly mixed, pour into the prepared cake tin and bake in the centre of the preheated oven for about 20 minutes (it should have risen and come away from the sides of the tin a little and a skewer inserted in the centre will come out clean when it is done). Allow to settle for a couple of minutes, then turn out on to a cooling rack. It might look a bit dry and wrinkled, but it tastes really good. As this cake contains wheat flour, try to make it an occasional treat.

Chestnut Sponge Cake

Makes one 18-cm (7-in) cake

1 large organic free-range egg
75 g (3 oz) unsweetened tinned
  chestnut purée
40 g (1½ oz) organic unsalted
  butter

50 g (2 oz) muscovado sugar
50 g (2 oz) cornflour
25 g (1 oz) potato flour
pinch bicarbonate of soda
pinch cream of tartar

Preheat the oven to 170°C/325°F and grease and line an 18-cm (7-in) cake tin. Break the egg into a bowl and add the chestnut purée. Beat until you have a smooth paste. In another bowl, cream together the butter and sugar. In a third bowl, sift together the flours and bicarbonate of soda and cream of tartar. Beat the egg and chestnut purée mixture gradually into the butter and sugar mixture. Fold the flour mixture into the creamed mixture and then tip it into the prepared cake tin. Bake in the preheated oven for 20 to 25 minutes, until risen and golden brown. Leave to cool in the tin for 10 minutes before turning out on to a wire cooling rack.

Potato Scones

Makes 12 scones

100 g (4 oz) cooked potatoes
2 medium organic free-range
  eggs, beaten
150 ml (¼ pint) rice milk
75 g (3 oz) ground rice
25 g (1 oz) lentil flour (also
  called gram flour)

25 g (1 oz) muscovado sugar
1 tsp bicarbonate of soda
pinch cream of tartar
50 ml (2 fl oz) olive oil

Preheat the oven to 220°C/425°F and grease a baking tray or bun tin. Beat the cooked potatoes with the egg and milk until a smooth purée forms. Mix all the dry ingredients together and add the olive oil. Fold the flour mixture into the purée. Spoon the mixture into small heaps on the preheated baking tray or bun tin. Cook in the preheated oven for 15–20 minutes, until brown.

DRINKS

Special Chamomile Tea

Serves 1

1 tsp dried chamomile flowers
1 strip orange zest
1 tsp honey
175 ml (6 fl oz) filtered water

Place the chamomile flowers, orange zest and honey in a teapot. Bring the water to the boil, then pour into the teapot. Stir well, then cover and leave to infuse for 8–10 minutes. Strain into a cup and serve hot, reheating if necessary.

Lemon Barley Water

Makes about 1.25 litres ($2\frac{1}{4}$ pints)

25 g (1 oz) pearl barley
1.2 l (2 pints) filtered water
zest of 1 lemon
120 ml (4 fl oz) fresh lemon juice
2 tsp raw honey or to taste

Place the pearl barley in a large saucepan and cover with a little of the water. Bring to the boil and simmer for 2 minutes, then strain into a clean pan. Stir in the lemon zest, juice and the remaining water and heat gently, stirring occasionally, until boiling. Reduce the heat, cover the pan and cook gently for 30 minutes. Leave covered until cold. Strain, sweeten to taste with the honey, then store in a covered container in the fridge for up to 1 week, using as required.

Cinnamon Tea

Makes about 1.5 litres (2½ pints)

2 cloves
5-cm (2-in) length cinnamon
  stick
1.2 l (2 pints) water

1 tbsp black tea leaves
50 ml (2 fl oz) orange juice
juice of 1 lemon
2 tsp raw honey or to taste

Place the cloves and cinnamon stick in a large saucepan with the water and bring to the boil. Pour this liquid over the tea leaves and infuse for 4–5 minutes. Strain. Add the honey to taste, then stir in the orange and lemon juices. Serve.

Fruit Smoothies

Serves 1

1 frozen banana (peeled and
  frozen), chopped
100 g (4 oz) of your favourite
  fresh fruit

250 ml (8 fl oz) apple juice for
  a thin drink or soya milk for
  a thicker drink

Place all the ingredients in a blender and whizz until well mixed. Serve.

Melon Reviver

Serves 1

½ galia melon, deseeded, quartered and peeled
2 pears, peeled and quartered
2.5-cm (1-in) piece fresh ginger root, peeled
filtered water as necessary

Place all the ingredients in a blender and whizz until well mixed. Add a little filtered water if required. Serve.

Citrus Shake

Serves 1

1 pink grapefruit, peeled and segmented
1 blood orange, peeled and segmented
2 tbsp lemon juice

Place the grapefruit and orange in a blender and whizz until well mixed. Add the lemon juice and serve.

Ginger Tea

Serves 2

300 ml ($\frac{1}{2}$ pint) filtered water
5-cm (2-in) piece fresh ginger root, peeled and sliced into very thin rounds
fresh lemon juice to taste
1 tsp raw honey, if required

Pour the water into a medium-sized saucepan. Add the ginger slices and bring to the boil. Boil for 5 minutes, then lower the heat and simmer very gently for 45 minutes. Strain the tea into cups and add lemon juice to taste. Add honey if required.

Carrot Smoothie

Serves 2

300 ml ($\frac{1}{2}$ pint) fresh carrot juice or 5 carrots, liquidized together with 300 ml ($\frac{1}{2}$ pint) filtered water

125 g ($4\frac{1}{2}$ oz) organic natural live yogurt
1 banana, peeled and chopped
3 fresh mint leaves (optional)

Pour the carrot juice into a blender and add the yogurt, banana and mint leaves, if using. Blend and serve.

Fruity Tango

Serves 2

1 apple, peeled and chopped
1 orange, peeled and
   segmented
1 banana, peeled and chopped

1 kiwi fruit, peeled and
   chopped or 6 strawberries
300 ml ($\frac{1}{2}$ pint) filtered water
3–4 ice cubes

Place the fruit in a blender and add the water and ice cubes. Whizz until smooth, then serve.

Banana Milk

Serves 1

1 banana, peeled and chopped
150 ml (5 fl oz) filtered water
$\frac{1}{2}$ tsp vanilla extract

Place all the ingredients in a blender and whizz until well mixed. Serve.

Useful Addresses

CFS Research Foundation
2 The Briars
Sarratt
Rickmansworth
Hertfordshire WD3 6AU
Tel: 01923 268641
Fax: 01923 260352

Supporting high-quality research aimed at understanding the basis of CFS/ME and its treatment.

Action for ME
PO Box 1302
Wells
Somerset BA5 1YE
Tel: 01749 670799
Fax: 01749 672561
Website: www.afme.org.uk
e-mail: admin@afme.org.uk

ANZMES Inc. (Action for New Zealand ME Sufferers)
PO Box 54-201
Bucklands Beach 1730
Auckland
New Zealand
Website: www.anzmes.org
e-mail: janice.roseingrave@xtra.co.nz

For CFS/ME information and support, either write or contact via the website or e-mail.

AACFS (American Association for Chronic Fatigue Syndrome)
515 Minor Avenue
Suite 18
Seattle
Washington
WA 98104
USA
Tel: 206 781 3544
Fax: 206 749 9052
Website: www.aacfs.org
e-mail: info@aacfs.org

Community Health Foundation
28 Wimpole Street
London W1M 7AD
Tel: 020 7636 5238
Fax: 020 7323 0698

For more information on the preparation of whole foods and classes on the principles and practice of macrobiotics (whole food diets that closely follow the pattern of nature).

West Bend Water Distillers (UK)
Tel: 740 544 5842
Website: www.water-distillers.com
e-mail: polarbearwater@aol.com
and
The West Bend Company
PO Box 2780
West Bend
Wisconsin
WI 53095-2780
USA
Tel: 262 334 6949
Website: www.westbend.com

Suppliers of water distillers.

Allergy and Environmental Sensitivity Support and Research Association (Australia)
PO Box 298
Ringwood
Victoria 3134
Australia
Tel: (61) 39888 1282

USEFUL ADDRESSES

The Soil Association
Bristol House
40–56 Victoria Street
Bristol BS1 6BY
Tel: 0117 929 0661
Fax: 0117 925 2504
Website: www.soilassociation.org
e-mail: info@soilassociation.org

The Nutri Centre
7 Park Crescent
London W1B 1PF
Tel: 020 7436 5122 (for orders of supplements)
Fax: 020 7436 5171
Website: www.nutricentre.com
e-mail: customerservices@nutricentre.com

For good-quality supplements and subscription to the regular *Nutri News* publication.

The Nutrition-Mission
PO Box 2
Cheltenham
Gloucestershire GL54 5YR
Tel: 01725 514222
Website: www.nutrition-mission.co.uk
e-mail: info@nutrition-mission.co.uk

For an excellent one-a-day high antioxidant containing over 30 ingredients, including the B vitamins and high-dose pantothenic acid and omega 3 and 6 essential fatty acids (which help to control pain), liver support (which gets the liver and gall bladder working properly so that toxins are expelled) and intestinal tone (which balances the gut flora and removes toxins from the body, helping to ease constipation or diarrhoea, flatulence and bloating).

BioCare Ltd
Lakeside
180 Lifford Lane
Kings Norton
Birmingham B30 3NU
Tel: 0121 433 3727 (for sales, orders and enquiries)
Fax: 0121 433 3879 (for sales and orders)
Website: www.biocare.co.uk
e-mail: biocare@biocare.co.uk

For magnesium malate (which helps reduce the pain and fatigue of CFS/ME) and sucroguard (which helps reduce food, sugar and cigarette cravings) and all other high-quality practitioner-grade supplements, including a one-a-day high antioxidant.

Bioforce (UK) Ltd
2 Brewster Place
Irvine
North Ayrshire KA11 5DD
Tel: 01294 277 344
Fax: 01294 277 922
Website: www.bioforce.co.uk
e-mail: enquiries@bioforce.co.uk

For healthy seasonings and so on.

Organics Direct
Olympic House
196 The Broadway
Wimbledon
London SW19 1SN
Tel: 020 8545 7676 (weekdays from 9 a.m.–6 p.m.)
Fax: 020 8545 7699
Website: www.organicsdirect.co.uk
e-mail: info@organicsdirect.co.uk

For fresh, organic produce. You can order online or by telephone and a brochure is available on request.

Nutricia
White Horse Business Park
Trowbridge
Wiltshire BA14 OXQ
Tel: 01225 711677
Fax: 01225 711812
Website: www.nutricia.com

and
Nutricia New Zealand Ltd
PO Box 62523
Central Park
Auckland 6
New Zealand
Tel: (64) 9 5700973
Fax: (64) 9 5700974
Website: www.babytimes.co.nz

For good-quality nutritional supplements.

Holland & Barrett
A chain of healthfood shops with branches throughout the UK.

National Association of Health Stores
Wayside Cottage
Cuckoo Corner
Urchfont
Devizes
Wiltshire SN10 4RA
Tel: 01380 840133

British Nutrition Foundation
High Holborn House
52–54 High Holborn
London WC1V 6RQ

Biotta Juices
Cedar Health Ltd
Pepper Road
Hazel Grove
Stockport
Cheshire SK7 5BW
Tel: 0161 483 1235
Fax: 0161 456 4321
Website: www.cedarhealth.co.uk
e-mail: info@cedarhealth.co.uk
and
Herbal Supplies Ltd
3 Jennifer Avenue
Ridgehaven 5097
Australia

For nutritious, organic vegetable juices in beetroot, celery, vegetable cocktail, carrot and Breuss varieties.

Pauls Tofu
Unit 9
66 Snow Hill
Melton Mowbray
Leicestershire LE13 1PH
Tel: 01664 60572

Supplier of organic tofu – an excellent substitute for dairy and animal products. Ring for a factsheet with recipes.

References

1 K. J. Pezke, A. Elsner, J. Proll, F. Thielecke and C. C. Metges (2000) *Journal of Nutrition*, **130**, pp. 2889–96.
2 A team of Japanese researchers, led by Dr Yoshiaki Somekawa. See (January 2001) 'Obstetrics and Gynecology' newsletter, **97**, 1.
3 A team of researchers, led by Dr Joseph Bellanti, carried out a placebo-controlled, double-blind study into the effects of Enada. See (February 1999), *Annals of Allergy, Asthma and Immunology*.
4 J. Kleijjnen (November 1992) *Lancet*, **340**, 8828.
5 D. Warot (1991) 'Comparative Effects of Ginkgo Biloba Extracts on Psychomotor Performance in Healthy Subjects', *Therapie*, **46**.
6 K. Kupparanjan, *et al.* (1980) 'Effect of Ashwagandha on the Process of Ageing in Human Volunteers', *Journal of Research in Ayurveda and Sadai*, pp. 247–58.

Further Reading

Martin Budd (2000) *Why am I so Tired?*, HarperCollins.

Trudie Chalder (1995) *Coping with Chronic Fatigue*, Sheldon Press.

Dr William G. Crook (1992) *Chronic Fatigue Syndrome and the Yeast Connection*, Professional Books.

Jill Dupleix (2002) *Simple Food*, Quadrille Publishing.

Donna Hay (2000) *Marie Claire Flavours*, Murdoch Books.

Patrick Holford (1998) *The Optimum Nutrition Bible*, Piatkus.

Leslie Kenton (2001) *The Raw Energy Bible*, Vermilion.

Dr John R. Lee and Virginia Hopkins (1996) *What Doctors May Not Tell You About Menopause: The breakthrough book on natural progesterone*, Warner Books.

Sharon Ann Rhoads (1978) *Cooking with Sea Vegetables*, Autumn Press.

Lorna Sass and Lorna J. Sass (1998) *New Soy Cookbook: Tempting recipes for soybeans, soy milk, tofu, tempeh, miso and soy sauce*, Chronicle Books.

Mary J. Shomon (2000) *Living Well with Hypothyroidism*, Harper-Resource.

Index